# From Sunset to Sunrise

Dorit Kreiser

D1607847

*This book is dedicated with love to my parents-Hannah and Shay, who loved, knew, and taught me how to sleep*

Producer & International Distributor
eBookPro Publishing
www.ebook-pro.com

**From Sunset to Sunrise**
**Dorit Kreiser**

Illustrations and Graphics by Pablo Boyanovsky Bazan
Cover Design by Orit Rubinstein
Review and Editorial Support: Avi Zechory, Blair O'Neil, Connie Nelson,
Cynthia Phillips, Meaghan Selger
Printed in the United States of America

Published by 1st Years Fundamentals www.atnightwesleep.com (Sleep
Book) www.sleepallnightusa.com (Sleep Consulting)

Contact: kreiserdorit@gmail.com
ISBN 9798596759549

# FROM SUNSET
# TO SUNRISE

*The Behavioral Method to Teach Children
Habits for a Full Night Sleep*

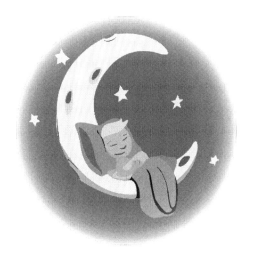

## DORIT KREISER

# Contents

Preface 11

Prologue 13

My Story 17

Wait! Why Do We Even Need to Sleep? 21

The Whole Theory in a Nutshell 25

The Parents' Job 27

Before We Start 30

The Unusual Age – When to Start Teaching a Baby to Sleep 33

The Method: "Shhh... at Night We Sleep" 39

Parents Must Sleep (and They Have the Right to) 47

Children Must Sleep (and they have the right to) 54

Fear of Abandonment 60

Goodbye to the Pacifier 64

Sleep...at the Mall 71

Baby Wants – Baby Needs 75

Food, a Bath, and to Bed 78

Breastfeeding or Formula – It's Not a Question! 98

The Baby Cried and Cried and Cried 105

In Practice – What Do We Do?                                    119

Fear Will Keep Mommy and Me Together                            149

Even When Sick – At Night We Sleep                              154

The "Tux" of the Method                                         160

Teething and Sleep                                              164

SIDS                                                            168

The Father's Role                                               173

Single Motherhood                                               176

My Daddy is the Tallest and My Mommy is the Prettiest          178

The Firstborn's Sleep                                           180

Siblings in the Same Boat                                       184

"Maybe"                                                         190

Implementing the Method – on a Flight                          196

Flying on Vacation – Who wants to come?                        202

Vacation and Sleep – It's Not a Problem                        205

A New Baby in the Family                                        208

Being an Excellent Parent is Dangerous                         210

Managing Daylight Savings Time                                 214

Old Wives' Tales                                                217

Sleep Training Vs Sleep Counseling                             219

When the Baby is Already Sleeping and You Aren't              223

Ugh! Regression                                               227

Sometimes You Need Help                                       229

Questions and Answers                                         231

Epilogue and Thanks                                           238

Appendixes and Addendums                                      241

# Preface

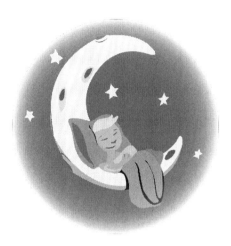

When I read Dorit Kreiser's book, I could only think one thing: How did I not have this book 25 years ago? As a doctor, I've spent many years sleep deprived – not only because of my long hours at the hospital, but also because I had three kids who did not know how to put themselves to sleep and continued waking up between sleep cycles. I would put them to sleep at night by feeding them or holding them in my arms. As they grew older, these methods became decreasingly effective. My family and I suffered from lack of sleep for years and, as a doctor, I understood the consequences of such deprivation well.

Back in the day, there were no sleep trainers nor books like the one written by Dorit, who I think of as a sleep fairy. I've known Dorit for more than 20 years. Her contribution to the world as a midwife, psychotherapist, parents' counselor and sleep trainer is incomparably grand. Dorit has been growing in practicing and teaching sleep training for years, and has made so many parents realize her field's importance. In her book, speaking in the first person form, Dorit clearly explains the scientific, historical, and personal background that led her to understand how crucial sleep is and develop the Shhh... at Night We Sleep method. She rightfully recommends that parents teach their babies how to sleep as early as the baby has a biological clock. The biological clock is fully developed by eight to twelve weeks after birth, at which point every baby should learn how to sleep. Dorit outlines how to achieve this goal in a friendly and clear manner. I loved Dorit's persistence in meeting each child's physical and emotional needs during the day, and teaching them how to sleep at night. Dorit has a great love for babies and children, but is also empathetic towards a parent's needs.

The book's readers will learn about humanity, human errors, and Dorit's insights and the unique Shhh...at Night We Sleep method. I am sure that anyone who will read the book and follow its recommendations and directions will enjoy the journey and consistently good nightly sleep.

**Irit Eisen, MD**
*Head of the Newborn Unit*
*The Haim Seba Medical Unit of Tel Hashomer*
*Israel*

# Prologue

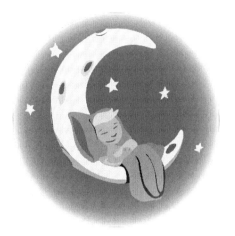

I have been asked to write this book so many times, and eventually, I could no longer refuse. Why did I hesitate? To be honest, I was afraid that a book would replace the wonderful work that I do with the many parents who have allowed me to help their families and touch their children's lives. I love these personal encounters so much that I was having a hard time with the idea that I would lose out on working with families one-on-one because people would only need to purchase and read my book.

Eventually, I overcame my concerns and I'm pleased to present a book with ideas and concepts that could transform your family's life. Yes, this is another book about how to help your baby sleep. There are lots of amazing books out there with great ideas and sound advice, but I have a different approach with my own clients:

I've developed a unique method that has helped thousands of babies around the world sleep through the night.

The method combines parental guidance with real milestones and dynamics that take place in children's day-to-day lives. I'll provide you with tools you can use during the day that will help your child at night. I've learned that what happens during the day has the potential to affect your child's sleep.

I've included all of my hard-learned parental mistakes to help you avoid them and to let you know you're not alone. Parenthood is not easy.

I truly believe that after you read this book and implement my method, your baby will sleep through the night. You will also experience a significant improvement in your quality of life without letting fear or rigid rules completely take over your parenting process.

My method addresses any problems that you may encounter that potentially interfere with sleep including teething, childhood illness, how to nurture sleep in unusual circumstances, and what to do when regression takes place.

It isn't simple being a parent. There are so many "methods" to teaching sleep, and so many different approaches. The abundance of options can create a lot of confusion. What method is right? Who is right? With so much contradicting research, who can be sure of the right way?

You've already tried so many things and so many methods. You've read everything that has been written, and nothing has worked. If only you could get your child to sleep with a smile and a magic wand.

This book is here to help you do something different and to assist you in teaching your baby one of the most important skills: S L E E P I N G.

After seven years as a certified midwife, I received a request from the hospital administration to run the soon-to-be opened maternity and infant ward.

The new ward was a success, but there was one problem – during the night shift, there were only three nurses caring for 30 babies, making it impossible to hold all of them –and all of them were constantly crying.

Mothers who came to visit their baby in the middle of the night were upset to find that their baby was left to cry.

I decided to investigate the issue and took a night shift.

I found devoted nurses who fed the babies on time, burped them, bathed them with care and kept them perfectly clean. I could not figure out why these healthy babies, who were so well cared for, were still crying. But, as I watched them, I noticed that the babies' crying slowly died down, and while making a particular motion with their hand each of them slowly closed their eyes and fell asleep.

"Wow…" I thought to myself. "Thanks to the fact that there was no one there to immediately pick them up, we gave them a chance to do it on their own."

I decided to investigate this discovery to figure out if it was a co-incidence or a phenomenon. I visited the ward night after night, and found that every single one of the babies put themselves to sleep after minutes of crying. Some took three minutes, some seven, and some even over thirty, but they all eventually put themselves to sleep and slept three to four hours (these were 2- to 3-day-old babies).

I started realizing that these newborn babies had not yet learned how to put themselves to sleep. While in the womb, they fell asleep along to their mothers' movements. From my time as a midwife, I can tell you that the baby usually moves in the womb when its mother is resting. I felt that I had discovered something very important.

Upon investigating literature on this subject, I realized that this was not an original discovery. A significant body of research shows that babies are born with the ability to self-regulate and self-soothe.

I then developed practices for parents to preserve and even strengthen their baby's ability to calm themselves down and to fall asleep. By preserving and strengthening the baby's congenital ability for self-soothing and calming, he or she can transition from one sleep cycle to the next, facilitating continuous sleep.

The only question that remained unanswered was whether it is okay for a baby to cry for minutes, or sometimes even longer. The benefits were clear to me, but I wondered if there was any harm in this practice. I spent five years studying two psychotherapy movements: Freud's psychodynamic therapy and Adler's individual psychology. When I was finished, I knew that I was ready to begin my journey.

I'm going to let you know in advance that my method might break a few myths, and you might feel that it's not the right thing to do during the first three days. Yet, after three days (on average), when your baby goes to bed and sleeps a full 10-12 hours uninterrupted, then wakes up in the morning full of energy and smiles back at you, you will understand that you made the right choice. Life isn't a sprint. Life is a marathon. I promise you that if you stick with my method, it will benefit both your baby and yourself.

After three days, your life could be like this:

It's 6 PM. Your baby knows the day is over. He or she will feel tired and will start getting ready for the falling-asleep process. He or she will be fed and bathed, instinctively knowing that the end of the day involves getting into bed for a sweet slumber. In bed, he or she will mumble to him- or herself for a few minutes, will do the 'soothing motion' (I'll talk more about this later) which will put him or her to sleep, and he will sleep through the night.

It isn't a dream. This could -- and should -- be your (and your child's) reality.

I hope you enjoy this book - I wrote it for you and your children. I wish you lots of success with the "Shhh...at Night We Sleep" method and many restful nights' sleep.

Yours,
**Dorit Kreiser**
*Founder & Master Sleep Coach At Night We Sleep*

# My Story

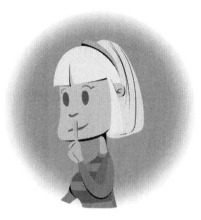

It's 5 AM—the hour our ancestors would wake up to hunt their first meal of the day. It's also the time that Shir, my eldest daughter, wakes up. I mumble to myself that she needs to eat. When I go to her room, she is as happy as a clam, the sweetest thing, smelling like something no soap company could ever replicate. I kiss her, breastfeed her, and burp her—and then she spits up everything she has eaten. Ugh! I try feeding her again because her stomach might be empty, but she refuses.

Half an hour later with no sleep, she's restless. I try to feed her again. I put her in bed, and she cries. I pick her up—I will not let my baby cry. She's almost asleep. I rock her, pat her, and success! Shir has fallen asleep. I stop breathing so I don't wake her. I put her in bed, but the transition from my arms to her bed wakes her. She is crying again. I decide to let her cry. Enough! I'm human, too. The crying turns into screaming. My mother's intuition whispers that it isn't right to let her cry. I pick up my precious baby, kiss her and tell her "Mommy won't let you cry, my treasure." It doesn't work. What the heck does she want from me? She ate, she played. I hugged and kissed her. I helped her fall asleep. What do I do with her now?

Plan B: the stroller. I rock her and sing her the lullaby that my mother used to sing to me. After singing it eight times, she's asleep. I leave her in the stroller, collapse on the couch and silently pray, "Please, dear God, give me just one hour of sleep." My princess sleeps for an hour and twenty minutes! It's a miracle. I take her out of the stroller, kiss her, and hug her.

This is what happens every time she is tired. Trying to get my daughter to sleep is like going to war. It's exhausting.

The day continues. We go for a stroll. We play. I make lunch. The moment I sit down to eat, she cries. I tell her, and myself, "Just a minute, honey, mommy has to eat." She screams.

I ask myself: what's more important, your meal or your daughter? I abandon my meal, pick her up, check her diaper, change her clothes so that she is nice and comfy, and put her to sleep.

She cries. I'm hungry. What do I do? I put her in her bouncer so that she can watch me eat. I take a few bites and she cries again. Is she hungry? Goodbye, lunch. I feed her. She eats like she hasn't eaten since she was born. I knew it! I always know what my baby wants. I am the best mother! She falls asleep in my arms. I am the perfect mom! Maybe I can sleep now. Then I see the laundry, and the grocery list, and the pregnancy test because I'm late. Yay.

I have no idea what to do so I call my mom. In an assertive and firm voice, my mother tells me that I have to rest, "When she sleeps, you sleep."

I listen to my wise mother's advice. Before I sleep, I do one load of laundry. Really quickly. I can't help myself. No rest for weary mothers. The moment my head touches the pillow she wakes up. Damn! And then a miracle happens, she goes back to sleep—another ten minutes.

I get ten minutes! I shut my eyes, and what does she do? She cries. It starts all over: Kiss, feed, burp, spit up. Then I hear the beloved sound, the sound of her father. My husband's car pulls up the driveway. He slept all night and 'hung out' with nice and interesting people at work all day, while I was barely able to find time for myself to go to the bathroom. He walks through the door and I hand him his daughter and say, "Take her! I didn't conceive her by myself!"

I feel a little guilty about being tired of my own baby and yelling at my beloved husband. I watch him as he laughs and smiles with her. He has it so easy, unlike me, who was at war with her all day. He gives her a bath while I load the dishwasher. Then it's time for pajamas, a goodnight ceremony with all her toys and her pacifier. We are both overwhelmed by her cuteness. Lights out. Then the mumbling starts, which turns into heart breaking cries. Her father goes to rock her in bed and puts the pacifier back in her mouth. It doesn't help, the crying only gets stronger. I come to the rescue to show my husband how it's done. I take her in my arms and sing the lullaby. It works! I take a deep breath and it wakes her up. I take shallow breaths. Who needs oxygen? At least she's asleep.

My husband asks me how I do it. In my superior mom mode, I say with a smug smile, "I know her."

Night. 2 AM. My smug smile doesn't last long. She's crying. I don't wake up. She screams. I get up, change her diaper, feed her—you know the drill. Nothing I do works.

AM. She cries. I don't get up. She screams. I can't get up. She screams until she almost chokes. I leap out of bed and apologize for being a horrible mother. Her clothes are drenched and her diaper is overflowing with poop. I'm completely overwhelmed by the disaster. I give her a bath and, finally, she sleeps, all thanks to the amazing care that Mother Dorit bestowed upon her daughter. I go to bed with a smile.

AM. The adrenaline surge of joy is so high, I can't sleep. Until, eventually, I do.

AM. The hour our ancestors woke up to hunt their first meal of the day. And the time my daughter Shir wakes up. The war begins again.

If my story sounds familiar to you, this book is for you. Putting a baby to sleep doesn't have to be a struggle. It doesn't need to include fear that a random noise will wake your baby. They need sleep just as much as you do. All you'll need to do is give your baby a kiss and a hug, say good night and put your baby in bed. And he or she will sleep. This is what will happen if you follow the step-by-step method of **"Shhh…at Night We Sleep."**

# Wait! Why Do We Even Need to Sleep?

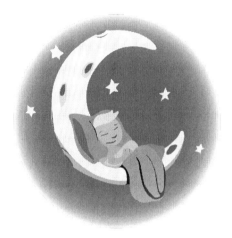

The question whether we need to sleep is, of course, a rhetorical one. We all know that we need to sleep. There are those who don't sleep enough hours due to unhealthy sleeping habits, there are those who suffer from physiological issues or daily stress, and there are those who don't sleep because their children don't know how to sleep through the night. Parents end up being "sleep aids" to get their child back to sleep because the child doesn't know how to transition from one sleep cycle to the next without parental help.

Sleep is essential for a healthy and enjoyable life. It supports our biological, cognitive, emotional, social and behavioral wellbeing. Sleep interruption and deprivation contribute to a slew of issues in many areas:

**Neurological:** During sleep the brain plays a significant role in recapturing data, in learning, and in memory processes, which all take place in the hippocampus area.

During the day, we interact with others and learn new skills. We will be better able to retain those skills the following day after a good night's sleep. For babies, there is a high degree of detachment from the stimuli-filled environment during sleep. Their sleep state simulates their time in the womb. This state facilitates physical rest, which promotes the maturing of the brain. During sleep, the brain is also working on processing the data from the day. There is clinical evidence that sleep during the early stages of a baby's life is necessary for brain development, physical growth, maturing of the immune system, regulation, maturing of many physical systems, and even the prevention of attention deficit disorders.

**Metabolic:** Sleep disorders and deprivation include risk of obesity, high body mass, high body fat and measurements, which can lead to the development of diabetes. Sleep also has an important part in body temperature regulation, metabolism and the recovery processes of the body and tissue.

**Endocrinology (Hormonal):** Sleep duration and quality have an impact on the neuro-endocrinology system, which explains observed stress responses in cases of chronic sleep deprivation. Sleep disorders are considered a stressor that causes a rise of stress hormones such as adrenaline and cortisol in the blood. High levels of the stress hormone cortisol during the evening hours can affect sensitivity to insulin the following morning. It also increases fat cells due to an increase of carbohydrate intake, which for many is a cause of fatigue. Sleep deprivation also causes a decline in the production of growth hormones. Secretion of the growth hormone reaches its peak level during the first half of the sleep process, and disruptions during this window of time impact hormonal functions.

**Immune System:** Sleep has an important role in healing processes and the functioning of the immune system. Severe sleep deprivation has been found to overly stimulate the immune system, just like stress does. In cases where the effects of sleep deprivation on the immune system were studied, it was found that sleep deprivation caused an elevation in granulocyte white blood cells, which elevate the inflammatory response.

---

### Did You Know?

*Over-secretion of cortisol from sleep deprivation can cause black under-eye circles and causes skin to appear tired and dull due to the prevention of collagen production, the protein responsible for plump and firm skin.*

---

**Circulatory System:** A decrease in sleep hours leads to an increase in blood pressure. A loss of half a night of sleep each week dramatically raises the risk of heart disease. Lack of sleep disrupts the peripheral blood flow, which affects the kidneys and blood pressure. Those who suffer from sleep deprivation have a higher probability of heart attacks compared to people who sleep an average of 8-9 hours a night.

**Personal and Social Life:** In a study comparing the cognitive performance of people who were sleep deprived with that of people who had consumed alcohol, the results showed an equal decrease in the psychomotor cognitive functioning in both groups. Sleep deprivation affects the entire family, including both the mother's state of mind and the relationship between parents and child. Mothers of babies who have sleep disorders have been found to suffer a variety of mental issues, including depression. Babies who don't sleep tend to cry more, and their restlessness and breastfeeding difficulties cause frustration on their parents' part.

### Did You Know?

*Your baby's high level of tiredness can manifest itself in apathy or sleepiness, or the opposite: excessive activity and overall restlessness.*

# The Whole Theory in a Nutshell

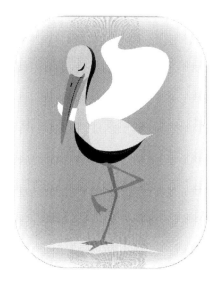

Parents always ask me: "So, what is this method of yours that teaches babies to sleep? Give me the whole thing in a nutshell."

In response, I usually tell these parents: "If you want your baby to learn how to sleep, put them in bed after a meal and a bath. When they're tired, just let them sleep."

A baby's sleep process takes about 15 to 30 minutes. During that time, the baby may mumble, move, complain and even protest being put to bed, especially after being cradled in its parent's arms. Even though it's much more pleasant for the baby to fall asleep in its parent's arms, he or she needs to learn to sleep on their own.

A baby must become accustomed to sleeping in his own bed.

Sleeping in his parent's arms for long periods of time is impossible and sleeping in his parent's bed can be dangerous.

Please do not expect your baby to be satisfied when you move him from the breast or from your arms into bed. Babies don't have to feel "content" at all times. For that reason, teaching my method 'in a nutshell,' would be to put your baby to bed after he's been fed, washed, and loved during the day. At night, just respond to him according to the method's instructions and teach him that at night we sleep.

In the following chapters, we will learn how to use the method step by step, and maybe even enjoy the process along the way.

Give your baby the credit that he or she can fall asleep and stay asleep.

The sense of capability may accompany him or her through life in other areas as well.

**YES, YOU CAN!**

# The Parents' Job

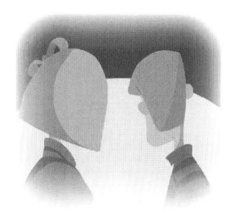

As parents, it's our job to care for our children's physical and emotional needs. In Abraham Maslow's Hierarchy of Needs, oxygen, food and sleep are defined as basic human needs.

A healthy baby can breathe on its own but can't make its own food. It also can't decide when to go to sleep or even initiate going to sleep on its own. As adults, we know what happens to us when we are hungry or tired; when we're hungry, we go to the fridge for food. When we're tired, we go to sleep. Babies need us for food, comfort, love and to teach them to sleep

Babies grow and thrive with two basic components:

1. **Nourishment** – A well-balanced diet to provide vital vitamins and nutrients the body can't produce on its own.
2. **Sleep** – The pituitary gland secretes the growth hormone, which among other things, is responsible for growth processes.

Many women understand the importance of breastfeeding, and to my great satisfaction, the number of women breastfeeding has been on the rise in recent years. Formula can also provide the necessary nutrients for your child. While there is an awareness of the importance of proper baby nutrition among parents and child development professionals, parents and professionals still lack awareness as to the importance of sleep on growth processes, development and health.

Self Fulfillment:
morality, creativity,
spontaneity, problem solving,
lacking prejudice, accepting reality

Respect & Admiration:
self esteem, confidence, success,
respecting others, respected by others

Sense of Belonging, Identity, and Love:
friendship, family, sexual intimacy

Physical Assurance:
of the body, work, resources, morality, family, health, belongings

Basic Physiology Needs:
oxygen, food, water, sleep, homeostasis, relieving

Sleep is important and essential for us all. It's especially vital for babies. Research notes that a third of babies and children suffer from sleep disorders, although my clinical experience indicates

a much higher percentage. Even parents who claim that their child has been sleeping wonderfully since the day they were born mean that he or she wakes up "only" three times to eat and goes back to sleep. While that may be completely normal for a 1- or 2-month -old, from the age of 3 or 4 months it is considered a sleep disorder, and not a "light" one at that. Sleeping issues with babies and children often appear subjective and thus parents interpret differently their baby's sleeping issues.

Ann and Jerry came to my clinic and told me that their 8-month-old baby Sue doesn't like to sleep and doesn't know how to put herself to sleep since she was born. They were sure that their baby had a medical condition. After I explained to them that falling asleep is a skill that babies need to learn and parents need to teach, they realized that doing so was within their capability and responsibility. They were very determined to succeed, and were very precise in their follow-through. Within three days, Sue learned how to put herself to sleep and slept 12 hours through the night.

They texted me: "Unreal!!! Sue is already sleeping 12 hours. This is the first time that we, too, slept through the night. Thank you, you are a true magician."

There are parents who decide to teach their child to sleep from the age of 3 months, and there are those who decide that the right time for their baby to sleep a full night is at the age of 12 months. It's possible to teach a baby to sleep at any stage that you decide is the right time. I recommend teaching babies to sleep as early as possible, and I'll elaborate more in upcoming chapters. I recommend that you make the decision that is right for your family after you read the book.

There are a lot of "experts" on social media and other parents and grandparents who are full of advice about how they put their kids to sleep. As I mentioned before, this can be a lot of white noise and it is important to follow the best sleep plan for you and your family.

As parents, we play a crucial role in influencing our child's sleeping patterns. I invite you to step outside of your comfort zone, as well as allow yourself to experience a certain level of frustration. I will walk you through a journey that you may find both interesting and exciting. Don't worry, we'll discuss parental rights later.

# Before We Start

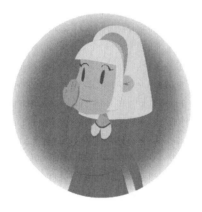

Before we start on this fabulous journey of teaching your baby or child to sleep, I want to clarify that there are cases in which there are medical reasons for waking up the baby during the night to eat, for limiting sleep time, or for delaying sleep training for a period of time. These medical cases are rare, and parents dealing with these issues are doing the best for their child. In the case of preemies (babies born before week 37), I recommend that you consult with your physician regarding the timing. There are other special cases that might prevent sleep training and may require a sleep coach.

This book is intended for parents of babies and children from 3 months to 5 year olds, who were born at full term (week 37 and on), at least six-and-a-half pounds at birth, and are diagnosed as healthy babies.

A few important facts to add:

1. Babies born after term (week 37 and on) develop better sleeping patterns than preemies which results in longer and restful sleep.

2. We humans are day creatures. Biologically, we need to be awake and active during the day and sleep at night. Thus, a newborn's brain is biologically predisposed to a preference for sleep at night and being awake during the day.

3. Today we live with the assistance of artificial lighting, which has brought extensive changes to our cultural and consumption habits, including changes to when we are awake and when we sleep. Yet our biological heritage remains the same.

4. Our sleep and wake patterns respond to light and darkness and through brain activity signaling us when it's time to sleep and when we should wake up.

5. You may hear comments such as, "A baby can only learn to sleep from the age of 5 months because only then does melatonin begin to be produced in the body." While it's true that during the first few months of a baby's life there are low levels of melatonin (the "darkness hormone" secreted by the pineal gland) present in the body, it doesn't mean that babies at this age don't need sleep and can't be taught this very important skill. To say it's impossible to teach a baby to sleep before the age of 5 months is like saying that a baby doesn't have the ability to breathe before that age. At 5-6 months, levels of melatonin increase with peak hormone secretion at night and are suppressed during the day. There is no link between this fact and the need and ability of a baby to sleep a full night from the age of 3 months. Melatonin levels reach their peak from the ages of 4 to 6, and from this stage a gradual decrease in its secretion occurs. This decrease continues as we develop, causing sleep disturbances in the elderly.

6. Studies indicate that the biological clock reaches maturity around three months of age and at this age, just like all human beings, babies that were born to term, should prefer eating during the day and sleeping at night.

7. My clinical experience has shown that the sooner a baby learns how to fall asleep on his or her own and sleeps through the night, parents have more patience for him or her during the day. Parents who have taught their babies to sleep say their baby is healthier and smiles more since learning critical sleeping skills in a healthy way.

> **Did You Know?**
>
> *Research indicates that sleep deprivation of as much as two hours a day could cause a decrease in brain function, lack of concentration, and an increase in accidents.*

# The Unusual Age – When to Start Teaching a Baby to Sleep

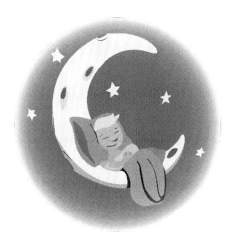

When is the right time to teach a baby how to sleep? One mother told me that she decided to come to me to teach her baby how to sleep after Googling "when to start teaching a baby to sleep" and getting a list of over 20,000 articles and opinions. When she looked for comfort in Facebook groups, she herself couldn't sleep at night because of all the confusion and countless differing opinions. The result is confused parents. While information is in abundance, we have to be sure it is based on reliable research.

In my opinion, babies should be taught how to sleep from the moment they are born. I can say that with proven results.

Chase's parents came to my clinic when he was 4 months old and weighed 14 pounds. When his mother started telling me about his sleeping habits, she burst into tears: "I can't handle it anymore. I am exhausted, and I feel bad for him too. He almost doesn't sleep during the day, and the longest that he manages to sleep during the night is between 9-11 PM. He is constantly on my breast, he calms down only on it, falls asleep for a few minutes. But I cannot stay still in that position."

Chase's father also looked tired and frustrated. He told me that while he does not breastfeed, he does wake up with his wife so that she will not be alone and he is afraid that she will fall asleep while holding the baby.

It was impossible not to feel their distress and frustration. This baby has two loving parents and the best type of food (breast milk), but is suffering from sleep deprivation, which is affecting his parents as well.

The only way I could encourage Chase's parents is by understanding them and giving them hope: "Today! Today, this is going to change. We will teach him the skill of falling asleep without depending on feeding. He will also be able to sleep for longer periods of time because he will be able to transition from one cycle to the next without the use of an external aid, which facilitates continuous sleep."

I gave them a lot of hope. To my great pleasure, Chase's parents followed the process very precisely and within only two days (!), he put himself to sleep and slept for a continuous 10 hours.

Two days later, he was having difficulty falling asleep again. They explained to me that they were out on a trip all day and that he fell asleep in the baby sling. I explained to Chase's mother that after a full day of falling asleep while being walked and rocked, his brain remembers and then he wants to fall asleep in the same way later too…. She understood, and when he was tired returned to put him back in the stroller, but with no rocking. She just let him fall asleep on his own.

Six months later, when Chase was 10 months old, they reported that he was still "sleeping like an angel... a full night. We got our lives back."

I don't teach babies to sleep for 10 hours straight through from day one, but I do teach them to fall asleep on their own between meals from their first day. We know how fast babies get used to falling asleep when they are held or only when they are rocked. Sleeping habits, the good and not-so-good, are set from the moment of birth. A newborn baby suckles, receives touch and love, and when he or she needs sleep, knows how to do it on his or her own. Food and sleep are basic needs and babies have a basic instinct to do both. We, as parents, can interfere with these skills from our own doing. We quickly habituate our baby to fall asleep on the breast or on the bottle or while rocking. Because a baby is learning from day one, it is the parents' responsibility to teach their baby basic natural skills and not acclimate him or her to habits which will work against them. A 2-month-old baby can learn and remember things for a period of two to three days. By consistently staying with the same method, your child can remember a habit for a longer period of time. At 2 months, you'll notice he or she doesn't like the bed, only wants the stroller, or wants to be rocked to sleep. Why does that happen? Because they remember from when they were infants. They remember being rocked to sleep or being put to sleep in your arms in the beginning. After that, they no longer agree to a change that is unfamiliar. So, if you've already accustomed your baby to only falling asleep in the stroller or only while riding in the car, this is the time to change those habits. On average, with my "Shhh... at Night We Sleep" method, your baby will adopt new habits within three days. And yes, for 3-month-old babies it can take only three days to acquire a new habit.

In breastfeeding, there is a chain of actions that need to be performed from the moment of birth, like placing the baby on the mother's nipple in order to 'awaken' the sucking reflex; to allow him or her to "open wide" so that the mouth presses on the entire areola and not just the nipple itself; and to stimulate the corners of the baby's mouth if he or she is unsuccessful in the sucking actions, etc. Sleeping skills need to be taught the same way, from the beginning.

Breastfeeding mothers should remember to breastfeed their infants according to their requirements, even if they do not sleep in between breastfeeding times, especially during the first 3 months, when the biological clock is not yet mature.

Every time your baby shows signs of hunger, please respond to it and feed your child. When feeding by formula, sleep patterns are more orderly, however it is still important to note that breastfeeding is the most preferable method of feeding your baby.

Some women don't succeed in breastfeeding, and not for lack of milk, which only happens in very rare cases. It's not because the baby doesn't want to eat, since there is no such thing. The main reason why some mothers don't succeed in breastfeeding is because they interfere too quickly with the natural process and disturb the baby's natural ability to suckle on its own, or they

don't teach the baby this skill when it becomes necessary. This is what should happen with sleep. A baby can sleep well from the moment of birth, and parents' over-interference in the process hinders the baby's natural ability to sleep. Parents think and expect that when you put a baby down to sleep, he or she should fall asleep within a few minutes. The falling-asleep process occurs in several stages, with the first stage from being awake to falling asleep taking about fifteen minutes on average. Parents who have intervened in the process from infancy need to change their interference and reteach the baby sleeping skills.

According to studies of the brain, as well as child psychology, the key time period for learning skills relatively quickly and easily is between birth and the age of three. This period is called "the critical period," during which brain cells develop quickly. Parents tend to think that it's best to wait to teach sleep until the baby "understands" or "communicates," but it turns out that these parents miss the most meaningful first years for learning.

During the early developmental stage, it is possible to teach babies and children almost anything. Their brains are exceptionally flexible, and new synapses and neurological connections are constantly created - like learning maps. Beyond the age of 3, these abilities decline significantly. Every baby can sleep—the success of this task depends only on the parents.

Dr. Suzuki, who was an educator post-WWII, developed a musical education method to imitate the way in which babies and children acquire their mother's language. If we accept the theory that language acquisition occurs naturally and that every human has the skill to acquire a language, we can also accept that any person can play an instrument in the same way that they can acquire language. The learning process is natural. Dr. Suzuki proved that it is possible to teach babies and young children how to play the violin in exactly the same way that they learned to talk. Furthermore, he claimed that every child can succeed and it all depends on the teaching method. Each time he lowered the age of the children that he taught, the child showed success in their studies. None of them was defined as a genius.

When you examine the early years of Mozart, the musical genius, for instance, you discover that his parents had an unusual awareness of musical education. Far be it for me to claim that Mozart was not a genius, but when I understand today what babies and children can be taught and I read about the invested educational process of Mozart's parents, particularly his father, I am not convinced that the secret here was his genius. What is clear is that from early childhood, Mozart was provided with the education and the environment required for making the absolute best of his talents.

I invite you, dear parents, to learn to take advantage of the never-ending ability of your children and to teach them anything you want. Let us start with the sleeping skill, because it is one of the basic needs and the foundation for your child's ability to learn additional skills.

The famous Japanese author Masaru Iboka writes in his book "Kindergarten is Too Late" that because the baby is so helpless, the abilities within him are great. In addition, he claims that while the brain of any newborn creature in nature is almost fully formed at birth, the brain of the human newborn is still Tabula Rasa (Latin for "blank slate"). The period during which the brain cells learn at the highest speed to create the nerve connections (synapses) is between birth and the age of 3. During the first six months following birth, the brain's capacity for perception reaches 50% of its full (mature-age) capacity. At the age of 3, it reaches 80%. The continued development during life is a function of the development until the age of 3.

Yet I still trust parents' intuition. Parents need to teach their children how to sleep when they think that it is time.

In the next chapter I write about the method I developed. I truly believe that the method is appropriate for all babies and all children, but like with any other method, it is not suitable for all parents. Let us embark on a journey of teaching your baby how to sleep with a behavioral method based on the baby's needs.

# The Method: "Shhh... at Night We Sleep"

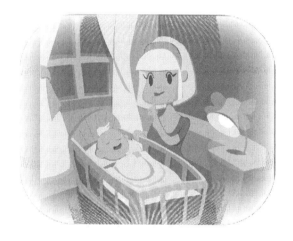

The "Shhh...at Night We Sleep" behavioral method is based on operational conditioning processes and classical learning. It isn't the "cry it out" system, but rather a system based on changing habits, eliminating bad sleeping habits, and relearning good sleeping habits, which will become automatic actions. Sleeping habits can be a curse as much as they can be a blessing. With the "Shhh...at Night We Sleep" method, we will create excellent sleeping habits for your child. And so you parents will also be able to go back to the way you used to sleep before you had a baby. Habits, as it turns out, are very powerful. They can cause our brain to stick with them while ignoring everything else, including reason.

Parents Emily and Gavin came to my clinic after hearing about my method sitting in a coffee shop. They spotted a couple sitting with a sleeping baby in a stroller for a full hour, despite the noise and commotion around them. They admired and complimented the couple, who replied: "Our Gordon is sleeping thanks to the 'Shhh…at Night We Sleep' method."

They asked for more details and found me.

They described Kim, their 10-month-old baby, and her inability to transfer from one sleep cycle to the next without a bottle of milk. They were exhausted, and said that the baby was constantly restless during the day as well as at night. They said that they performed a bedtime ritual and tried to put her down in her bed, but that she woke up every 60 to 90 minutes – and this has been going on for the past ten months.

Our session took place via Skype because they lived far from my clinic.

On the first day, they experienced great difficulty because Kim was "addicted" to the milk bottle. Despite their difficulty, they wanted to be 100% accurate and follow the process. They tended to her according to the method, and also learned when it was not right to interrupt her learning-to-sleep process.

The result: within three days, the child slept eleven and a half hours straight through and woke up with a big smile.

After the third day, they reported back in amazement, "You know, before we even got to you, we essentially did 80% of what you told us to do, but the little changes that we made following the instruction of the method are the ones that got our baby to sleep through the night."

Even little changes can put an end to a problematic sleeping pattern and create excellent sleeping habits. When you help your baby create good sleeping habits, you will be surprised at the other good habits they develop. Research indicates that when one good habit is created, it brings on the development of additional good habits.

That is what 3-year-old Michael's parents told me. Michael learned how to sleep on his own in his own bed, and subsequently improved his behavior in daycare. The teachers reported that he became more social and was more focused during learning sessions. It was easier to get him to clear his plate from the table, which was something he refused to do before his parents started sleep training. When I told his parents that there was a good chance that their child was behaving better due to sleeping better, they wholeheartedly agreed, because it was obviously easier for their son to learn new positive habits after sleeping better.

The "Shhh…at Night We Sleep" method allows the child to put itself to sleep with consistent parental assistance until he or she finds the motion that soothes them, what I call the "transitional motion," an analogy to Donald Winnicott's "transitional object."

Some parents think that there are only two approaches to teaching babies how to sleep: A, let the baby cry, or B, stay with the baby until it falls asleep.

Both are wrong! Even parents who think they have to stay close to their children and help them sleep also want children who have higher focusing abilities, better moods, and an easier time learning new things. To achieve all of the above, your children have to sleep a full night consistently. Consistency is very important.

When I wanted to lose ten pounds, I tried all sorts of methods. I separated protein from carbs, I cut out carbs, I ate only carbs, I ate a balanced diet of protein, fat and carbs, I cut out sugar, I cut out gluten, I combined diet with exercise. Nothing helped. If I lost weight with one of these plans, I quickly gained it back after a special event during which I only "tasted" a few desserts. What can I say? It isn't every day that a friend marries off a daughter. None of the "eating plans" I tried actually turned into a habit for me.

I only succeeded when I chose a method and stuck with it. I didn't let any message boards on the internet sway me from my goal. I didn't let unsubstantiated research affect my decision or my actions. Once I made a decision regarding the right method for me (and followed it carefully), I lost eight pounds. I left myself two as a souvenir.

The first week was hard, but to this day I stick with it. I don't care that there are friends who say that I have lost some of my "joy for life," and I don't care what different dietitians write about this specific diet. I chose it and it turned into a habit for me. I admit that occasionally I stray from it. I'm human. You will learn that in the "Shhh…at Night We Sleep" method there is room to break the routine as well. Despite the strong connection between food and sleep, let's return to the issue at hand: teaching your baby to learn to sleep.

An additional important element related to the "Shhh…at Night We Sleep" method is the changing of habits that the child has acquired from birth. With this method, we take advantage of babies' ability to quickly acquire new habits. How does the method work so fast? The origin of the answer is in the basic nucleus of our brain. It turns out that basic nuclei play a major role in memory of patterns and actions. In other words, basic nuclei store habits even while the rest of the brain goes to sleep. According to scientists, habits are formed because the brain is always seeking to exert the least amount of effort. If we leave it be, the brain will attempt to turn almost any routine action into a habit, because habits allow our brain to cut back on its activities more often. The natural tendency of conservation of energy is a huge advantage. Bad sleeping habits in babies and children can be changed or replaced with others. It is important to know that when a habit is formed, the brain stops working as hard, or it diverts the focus to other tasks. If we don't object purposefully and don't suggest other routine actions, the pattern will automatically exist. And it's the same with your child's sleeping habits. If we don't do something else and transition to a new, healthier, and better routine, the problematic sleep pattern will persist. In the "Shhh…at Night We Sleep" method we work on new routines. No more putting the baby to sleep in your arms, while driving or taking a stroll at night.

If I were reading a book like this, I would immediately look through the table of contents for the method and get right to it. I have no patience for the superfluous. I want to do the right thing right away. But in this case the background and explanations are very important, which is why the system is embedded within the different chapters. I want to make things easier for you. I want this book to be a professional guide loyal to a system that requires determination, consistency and accuracy. Without knowing and understanding the theories around the development of this method, you will have a harder time implementing it. If you read the book page by page and implement the method, you will be able to get to a place where your baby will sleep a full ten to twelve hours straight through the night within an average of three days.

My late grandmother, Ganesia Rabina, used to quote the 18th century Swiss philosopher Jean-Jacques Rousseau: "Patience is bitter, but its fruit is sweet."

Please wait patiently, and read every chapter. I hope this book will be like that person you meet on the street who gives you advice, or a movie you watched that changed your outlook and your quality of life.

I developed this method from years of serving as the head nurse in the newborn ward at a maternity hotel, where new mothers would stay during the first few days after giving birth. There, I observed babies who were well-fed, bathed and tired, and then put to sleep but were unable to fall asleep. Instead of closing their eyes and falling asleep, they fussed and cried. Sleep took a few minutes to a few hours.

I noticed that when parents attempted to help their babies sleep by putting a pacifier in their mouth, picking them up, or sticking a nipple in their mouth, their babies calmed down for a very brief period, but then went back to crying because they were tired. Some of the babies refused to take the pacifier, some moved their head away from the nipple because they were not hungry, and some just kept crying even in the parents' or the nurse's arms. The parents stood helplessly with their crying baby in their arms, when in fact they didn't understand that the baby would keep crying until it was put in the crib and allowed to get what it needed most…sleep! A baby needs touch, but not when it needs to sleep.

When babies were placed in the care of the nurses and put to sleep after a meal and a bath, they cried for a while, but the nurses were too busy with the other babies and were not able to cradle them to sleep in their arms and sing a lullaby. When the babies were in their own cribs, they were able to calm themselves down within a few minutes with motions they made with their hands.

I studied this motion for an entire year, until I knew that I had discovered what babies need to do to develop their independent sleeping skills - and how this skill is often affected by parental intervention. These observations are in line with theories of classical learning and operational conditioning. It was then that I truly understood how a baby is born with the ability to sleep and what parental intervention can do, for better or for worse.

There is a known saying in medicine that it's more important for a doctor to know what not to do rather than what to do. It's the same with the sleeping process of babies and children. My method is behavioral; based on learning and behavioral theories, and on parental determination and consistency. It includes what parents should do, and mostly what they should avoid doing. These are the things that every baby needs for growth and confidence in the world and in themselves.

Parents shouldn't be strict with their children about this, just to be consistent.

Babies are born with the sensory understanding of pleasure and act according to it. Sigmund Freud's theory describes pleasure as the principle that drives the human being from the moment he or she is born – ultimately intent on maximizing pleasure and minimizing pain and suffering. This action is called the 'Id,' which is the subconscious part of the soul. The pleasure which Freud speaks of is mostly biological-physical. Thanks to this method, your baby will learn how to sleep. Parents won't interrupt the process of falling asleep to pick up the baby at a time when he or she wants to be horizontal and fall asleep. That is the reason why babies, who learn how to sleep according to the method, sleep a full night after an average of three days, and not after weeks or months. After proper sleep training, the baby feels good about sleeping, it becomes a pleasure. Parents guide the child to move from one sleeping cycle to the next without interruption and so he or she sleeps better.

There are two themes in the "Shhh…at Night We Sleep" method:

1. We are the parents here.
2. Now it's nighttime and it is time to sleep.

When you identify with and embody this message, it will transfer to your baby. Through this method, we do what the baby needs, not what the parent feels. We don't allow emotional considerations. What parents think and feel is very important, but what guides parental behavior in this method is what the baby needs. The baby needs to sleep, and that is the ultimate goal. The How is very simple. Put the baby in bed, respond to him or her methodically and consistently with determination. This applies to 3-months-old babies to childhood. You are going to feel excited about the change which will occur in your child's sleep and in yours, as well as additional "side effects," such as a calmer child who smiles more, and a better relationship between you and your child.

The definition of the word "method" is a set order of an action or several actions performed to solve a certain problem.

Similarly, the method behind "Shhh...at Night We Sleep" consists of actions which you, the parents, need to make to resolve the issue of your baby's sleep. As with any method, this method has an order of actions and a set of very clear and strong ideas that need to be followed.

# Parents Must Sleep
# (and They Have the Right to)

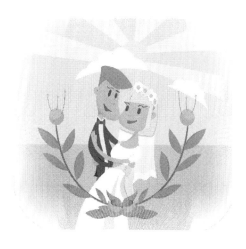

By the time I turned 23 I was already a mother of two, with a 22-month difference between the two. Everything was easy with my children. They were sweet, smiley, and fit every expectation that I had as a young mother. They were crawling on time, reaching out their hands to a toy even before the developmental nurse said they should, and gaining weight "nicely" (as one of the grandmothers used to say). Only one thing was unbearable (to say the least): they didn't sleep well. Neither one of them knew how to sleep. My eldest, Shir (who you've already met) would only sleep in my arms with a lullaby until she was 2 years old. Itay, my son, only screamed. It wasn't possible to get him to sleep even in my arms. The only days that I felt rested while they were young were when my wonderful sister would come to help me, or when I sent them for a sleepover at their Grandma Pearl and Grandpa Jacob's house.

When I got eight hours of uninterrupted sleep, I had all of the energy required to play on the rug with them, build a Lego tower, and work with playdough. On those days, I was the perfect mother because I myself had slept through the night. The following day, I couldn't stop thinking about the day before, how wonderful it was, how peaceful the house was. I asked myself what happened the previous day that was absent in the next. The answer came rather quickly – a good night's sleep. Until I got the rest I needed all I wanted to do was sleep, while after a full night's sleep, I came to a realization that I carry with me to this day:

**We, the parents, must sleep**. We have to sleep to function properly, to be better people and more productive for ourselves, and, mostly to be better parents. And you know what? It's also our basic right. Our children aren't aware of our basic needs, which is why we are the ones who need to make sure that these needs are met so that we can patiently and responsibly take care of our children.

The night that I first slept a full night as a mother was a turning point in my parenthood. I realized that when I take care of my own needs and my physical and emotional welfare, I can give more of myself than when I put aside everything that I need as a person and as a mother. I realized that if I don't sleep at night, I am irritable and less pleasant with my husband, my children and everyone around me. I don't have the energy reserves required to provide them with quality time, love and everything that they need from me during the day, and I can't enjoy what life is offering me either. In those days, pleasure had no part of my life. Life was survival. I recall the ambivalence that I experienced. What? I can't take a nap. Who will prepare supper? (I wanted to be a good wife). I can't rest. I have to do the laundry and pick up the children's toys. I should take her out for a walk in the park and let her experience nature, people, and stories. I saw everyone's needs, but my own.

Don't get me wrong - all in all, I was a happy person, but a very tired one. I felt like an empty pitcher, you expect to pour water out only to find out that it is empty. To be a good mom, I realized that I had to start sleeping well, no matter what. There was no internet back then, I couldn't Google "sleep coach," and there weren't any books available to guide me on how to put my baby to sleep. The only thing that I could do, and did, was go to the pediatrician and tell him that apparently there was something wrong with my children.

I told him: "They constantly cry in bed and only fall asleep in my arms or in the stroller. They wake up two to three times each night, and at different times."

I admit that in those days my focus was on my hardship and tiredness. I was unaware of the physical and emotional damage to my children because they weren't sleeping a full night.

The doctor said, "Let them eat every time they wake up, then they'll sleep."

I followed his instructions, and it only got worse. They would get up to eat, in some cases they would throw up, and want to fall asleep in my arms. I found myself not sleeping at all. I didn't want to wake up my husband because I knew that he needed to wake up early and drive through heavy traffic to a challenging workday. I didn't want to take the chance that he would have an accident due to lack of sleep. I didn't know what to do. I was exhausted. I was functioning on the most basic level.

Then we decided that apparently, in order to sleep, one must pay. My husband and I were only students with a very limited budget, but I decided to call a private physician who at the time was head of the pediatric ward at a nearby hospital.

She examined them from head to toe, and said to me: "Dorit, your children are perfectly healthy. They are crying for one reason only. They are tired and they have bad sleeping habits."

She suggested that I stop feeding them at night because it adversely affects the sleep process and they don't need food at night. She then gave me another golden piece of advice: separate rooms. The house we lived in was small. I told her that we didn't have an extra room. She started walking around the house and went into my study, and saw that there was enough room to put Itay's crib in the room. Having no other choice, we did as she said. It didn't feel right that the baby, my little prince, should sleep in the study, but I was desperate and ready to try anything. We moved the desk and moved in his crib and I stopped feeding him at night, and ever since then, he slept through the night. Just like that. For years I was thankful to the doctor every morning after a peaceful night of sleep. Until her visit to our home, I didn't know what sleep was. With Shir, my eldest, the process was more difficult and took longer because she wouldn't give in. She was in her terrible twos. As a young parent, I didn't know that I shouldn't have engaged her and I didn't know how to get out of it, so I just surrendered and did what she wanted, which was to fall asleep only in my arms and then for us to sleep with her, and then a bedtime story, and then just another last one, and then the pacifier... it was never-ending!

My labor pains were quickly forgotten, but I will never forget the sleep deprivation. With Rona, my third child, born after I had slept well for eight years – things were different. I taught her how to sleep on day one. In the first 3 months, I fed her. When I observed that the food was just getting in the way at night and she really didn't need it, I taught her to detach the link between eating and sleeping. I didn't let her fall asleep on my breast or a bottle. I made sure that I fed her when she was fully awake. If she attempted to fall asleep while suckling, I immediately softly tickled her cheek. She would smile and continue to eat without falling asleep during feeding. When she woke up during the night I would still make the usual mistake of picking her up "just for a minute" of hugging and kissing. I was unaware of the fact that I was interfering with her sleep process.

What a pity it is that I discovered the secret of how to teach babies how to sleep after she had turned 2. Later, when I observed as the head of the infant ward, combined with my knowledge in education, I started helping my friends and their babies with how to sleep and the process was successful 100% of the time. That was it! Bingo! I realized that I had stumbled upon an ingenious solution. There was only one problem.

Sometimes the method involved crying. Crying to me meant suffering, and there was no way that I would let my daughter or my friends' children cry…and if I did, then for how long? What were the ramifications? Babies should grow up in bliss. They can't hurt. They can't be caused any suffering. They should feel that they were born into a good and safe world. So what do we do?

My intuition told me that it wasn't too terrible if the babies cried a little. Babies cry for all sorts of reasons, including being tired when they are in our arms. At least then we hold them in our arms so our conscience is clearer. I didn't want to deal with my conscience.

The truth was that everything was clear to me except for the issue of ignoring the crying. One of the babies I had observed had cried for a minute and a half and then fell asleep, another had cried for twenty minutes, and a third went all out and cried for thirty-five minutes straight.

Then a good friend of mine, Talya, whose daughter Maya was 4-months old at the time, said to me: "Do with my Maya whatever you want before I return her to the maternity ward! And yes, I no longer care how much she cries because she doesn't stop crying even in my arms, even on the swing, and I am exhausted."

If my friend, the best and most sensitive person on earth, says she no longer has a problem with her baby crying as much as is necessary for her to learn how to sleep, I realized what was making people lose sleep.

I thought about what Talya had said. If at night they cried a little during the process of falling asleep, then that was okay. I understood that babies cry anyway, even when they are in your arms. They cry because they are tired and no method will soothe them in the long run. There are cases in which rocking or holding them in your arms will calm them down, but only for a short time. When they are in transition into the deep sleep phase and the parents put them back in bed, they wake up again and cry. Parents react inconsistently. Sometimes they try to rock, sometimes they pick the baby up in their arms, other times they give him a pacifier. If the baby rejects it, they buy a special pacifier for refusers. I realized that crying is their way of expressing tired frustration and the way to minimize their level of tired frustration is to let them sleep.

Our outlooks may differ. The outlook regarding the sleep of children in this book is different than some of the more prevalent ways of thinking. The method and I are not superior to other acceptable practices. If there are things that you disagree with, that's okay. I will be content if you only read this book with an open mind to a unique and different approach, and at the end you can decide if you want to go for it or not. Try to set aside the familiar, and dare to open up to new ideas.

At the end of the book you will find my contact details including my website, where you can discover a variety of current research regarding the processes and skills to teach babies and children different approaches to eating and sleeping.

Before we continue this journey, I would like to inform those parents who have not been convinced that it is their duty to sleep of the ramifications of sleep deprivation in adults:

- Attention disorders
- Physical and mental manifestations simulating inebriation
- Automobile accidents
- Endless quarreling (with spouses and others)
- Lack of concentration
- Lack of patience and tolerance
- Increased risk of mistakes at work
- Adult onset diabetes
- Cancer
- Autoimmune diseases
- Obesity
- Heart disease

If all this didn't convince you that you should sleep, then maybe you should read the chapter on why children should sleep…

# Children Must Sleep
## (and they have the right to)

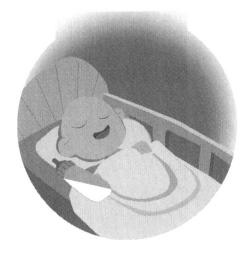

At the base of the Hierarchy of Needs (mentioned earlier) is food and sleep. Just as babies cannot live without food, they cannot live without sleep.

Many parents say, "My baby doesn't like to sleep," or "My baby doesn't want to sleep," or "Our baby is very alert."

But these sayings are, in fact, equivalent to the parent saying: "My baby doesn't like to breathe...or doesn't need to breathe."

All babies have to sleep from day one (they even sleep in the womb). It is only because there are changes in the baby's age and the number of hours that its stomach can hold food that parents experience confusion and uncertainty.

So let's set things straight:

Babies who came to term (born week 37 and on) at a weight of at least six-and-a-half pounds and are defined as healthy babies, should sleep almost the entire day and night, except for feeding and bathing time. They will usually eat every 2-4 hours and sleep in between. All of this will happen up until the age of 3-4 months.

From the age of 3-4 months, they are expected to nap about three times a day (an hour-and-a half each time) and at night we expect them to sleep about 10 hours nonstop. There are parents who have used my method who reported 12 hours of nonstop sleep.

For babies who were born prematurely (before week 37) or babies with health issues, there are other medical directions that need to be followed. For those, I recommend personal coaching and close supervision.

Many parents turn to counseling and sleep coaching for their baby because they are already exhausted. There are those among them who are concerned with their baby's sleep deprivation, but most parents still come because they feel frustrated, unfocused and tired day and night.

**Sleep disturbances and sleep deprivation in babies can cause one or more of these symptoms:**

- Attention disorders
- Diminished focusing and concentration ability
- Psychomotor restlessness / hyperactivity
- Developmental delays
- Slowing down of growth (weight and height)
- Diabetes
- Autoimmune diseases
- Constipation and digestive problems
- And more…

If you haven't been successful in teaching your baby to sleep a full night with or without assistance, you need to do **something different**.

> **"If you want something you have never had, you must do something you have never done."**
>
> *– Albert Einstein*

I would like to invite you to take the path, which I have found to be the most effective, safe and professional way to teach your children to sleep through the whole night.

In their book "Change: Principles of Problem Formation and Problem Resolution" Paul Watzlawick, John Weakland and Richard Fisch state that the worst way to find a solution to a problem is to do "more of the same."

That is why, if this time you want to achieve different results than those you have achieved, you have to do something that you have never done before.

When there is a clear and logical goal, the "how" should be goalfocused. That is what this book will do: Help you act towards the noble cause of your baby sleeping through the night.

Life often provides us with an undesirable reality. This can include health issues, divorce, accidents, and all sorts of obstacles. Sometimes with children come horrible realities, like a severe illness, or the need to undergo an operation....A child might have to deal with his or her parents getting a divorce, or, the worst could happen—a child might lose a parent. Of course, there are endless inconceivable and painful tragedies, especially for a young child who has just started life.

How is all of this related to sleep?

In cases of an undesirable reality, there are things that children must do or go through, even if it breaks our hearts.

The process of teaching how to fall asleep is not always an easy one. Babies who have been accustomed to falling asleep in a parent's arms or in the stroller will have a hard time changing those habits. Most babies are held when they are breastfed or bottle fed, and they are placed closely to a parent or another significant adult during the day.

When they find themselves on a firm mattress and not in the soft arms of mom or dad, they are all of a sudden in an undesirable reality. A baby needing to detach and move into a bed will not accept it with joy and pleasure. As far as the child is concerned, this is a downgrade in terms and conditions.

But just like in other situations in life when there is an undesirable reality and one needs to learn how to deal with it, the child needs to learn that this is a situation in which the day ends and he or she need to sleep on their own.

This is a task that a baby or a child can (and should) do on their own, but this moment during which they are put in bed is an unenjoyable one.

The crying that begins within seconds is as like the child saying to his parents, "I'm not having fun. It's better that I stay in your arms and you cradle me, or take me in the stroller out on the sidewalk where there are bumps which make it feel like a rocking chair and then sleeping is more fun."

They are having a hard time parting from the wonderful day that they had just had. They played, received attention, love and touch, and the parents were there for them or they were placed in a daycare center filled with friends and toys and a caring teacher. To go into a dark room in the evening hours and to part with all of this fun is not a simple task.

They want more. They want their parents close to them, because that's more fun. Remember the principle of pleasure; children will make any effort to increase pleasure. The tool through which they express their discontent is crying.

When children cry while getting shots, the parents don't like the crying. But, of course, they say: "There's no choice. You have to get the shot."

That is exactly what you will have to say to your child when he or she needs to go to sleep. There is nothing that can be done! You have to sleep! A child needs to learn how to cope with unwanted realities at any age. The undesirable reality, in this case, is just that the baby needs to part with the day and his parents in order to go to sleep. A baby who doesn't experience frustration at infancy will not be able to handle challenges during childhood, a deficiency that they will then take into adulthood.

As a midwife, I can tell you that babies deal with an undesirable reality from the moment they are born. While still in the womb, when labor begins, there is a decrease in blood flow to the womb and the baby is required to go through a short "boot camp" and deal with stress. The process of experiencing undesirable reality continues with the extraction of the head and the shoulders during normal vaginal birth, and especially when there is a need for mechanical aids. Immediately after, the baby is placed in a cool, well-lit room and covered in hospital sheets. Then the baby is taken for a series of tests, poked, probed and so on.

This is not a pampered journey. The frustration and discomfort the baby experiences are unavoidable. **In fact, they are essential to their health and development**. From the moment of birth, a baby must learn to deal with age-appropriate frustration, and its ability to deal with these frustrations allows it to grow and develop. Judith Viorst writes in her fabulous book "Life" about the necessary links between loss and the gains that we derive from it. The book talks about the things one gives up on in order to grow. She brilliantly describes how we start the process of giving up on things as early as the first years of our lives, in order to grow into independent people of the future.

So, a baby **must sleep** and it doesn't matter if he or she wants to or if it involves temporary separation difficulties from the parent or from the wonderful day which preceded the night. One does what is required in life, and **sleep is required**. As a rule, I prefer when raising children is done according to their needs, and parents have the responsibility to provide them with their needs.

# Fear of Abandonment

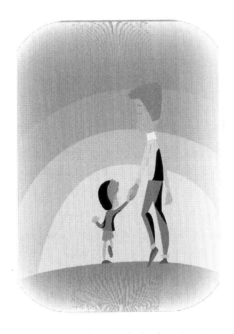

When parents start treating their baby's sleeping issues, they are pre-occupied with only one question – what the baby wants — and not what the baby needs. One of the questions that parents ask me is, "What will happen if I put my baby down to sleep and he will not want me to leave his room but I do leave the room? Will he develop fear of abandonment?"

I feel that it's important to clarify the term, because I encounter parents using it incorrectly.

Michael's parents came to see me when he was 9-months old.

"Please help us," they said, "before we are so tired that we divorce." Michael had not slept one full night since the day he was born.

I understood where they were coming from and I know exactly what tiredness does to people in general, and to couples in particular.

I asked them all the questions about Michael's and their habits, and then I explained the process, to which Michael's father said: "Wow... I am concerned that if he is in his bed and we are not right next to him he might experience fear of abandonment."

I asked him if he felt that he is an abandoning parent and he smiled and said: "Not at all, we are loving and devoted parents."

I explained that fear of abandonment at Michael's age is part of a normal developmental process. When they go to the bathroom or the kitchen for a moment, the child seeks them, and that is preparation for his ability to know how to remain with a sense of security even when he is alone. Fear of abandonment does not occur due to crying or to staying in your bed for the purpose of continuous sleep, especially when the process takes only three days on average.

Michael's mother shared that this explanation was important to her and that now she could understand why he cries when she leaves him for a moment to bring a bottle or a diaper. This is referenced in Donald Winnicott's important article about a baby's ability to be alone, which is a very important skill in the context of love and safety. Fear of abandonment is a psychological condition in which a person experiences fear resulting from a separation from an object or a person, child or adult, whom they have an emotional connection to, such as a house, mother, or father. This fear is prevalent amongst babies and young children and constitutes a part of their proper development. When it appears at later ages, and in cases where the fear is elevated or adversely affects the person's proper functioning, it is called "Separation Anxiety Phobia."

Babies who are used to having their parents next to them 24/7 could be susceptible to experiencing difficulty in parting with their parents for kindergarten and older grades. In extreme cases, there is a pathological fear of abandonment when there is a lack of a consistent figure in the child's life. This anxiety is never caused by a child's process of learning to sleep.

There are those who claim that from the age of 6 months to 2 years (when the permanent parental figure is internalized), if the parental figure suddenly disappears for more than four consecutive nights then there is a risk that the child will experience this separation anxiety and the relationship with the parent is threatened. Fear of the parent leaving without returning sets in, and it takes about four weeks until the child regains trust in his parents.

Some parents fear (and wrongly so) that teaching a baby to sleep might cause separation anxiety, but nothing in what happens when the parents put their baby to sleep after a day filled with activities, love, play and touch, or in requiring their baby or child to go to bed (thus allowing him or her to fall asleep on his or her own) can cause a pathological fear of abandonment. It's natural if parents are not present during the day and only see their child in the evening, that the parents could interpret their baby's crying when transitioned to bed as fear of abandonment.

This is where I would suggest to those parents to reevaluate. Look into whether they had enough time with their child and whether the child's basic physical and emotional needs were met during the day. At night there is no time or room for fulfilling any need but sleep. Night isn't the time to do with the child what was expected of the parents to do during the day.

In his article The Capacity to be Alone, Donald Winnicott claims that the ability to be alone is one of the most important factors of emotional maturity and the basis to build mature relationships. The ability to be alone does not negate the ability to be in a relationship. Naomi Zoran, PhD., a clinical psychologist, says that when you teach a baby to sleep, the only anxiety is the transferring of the anxiety of the parents onto the child.

Some parents are unaware that when they do not remove themselves from their child's presence when he or she is sleeping, the parents are in fact the ones who are experiencing anxiety. The baby just needs to sleep. When I identify that the parents are experiencing anxiety, I try to get to the root cause and deduce how it is possible to treat their anxiety without passing it on to their child.

The parents' anxiety is increased when they encounter negative reactions from the baby (a natural reaction to experiencing change), for example, when the parents are away on vacation.

Parents, you are allowed to go away on a couple's weekend and put your child's care in the loving arms of someone else, such as their grandparents. Even if you are not greeted with a huge smile by your children when you return, you will have to be understanding. Allow them the time required to adjust to your return and the smiles and love will soon resume as well. The children will benefit from getting back two happy parents - a couple of parents who took the time they needed together to strengthen their relationship, which is the basis for a positive atmosphere at home.

# Goodbye to the Pacifier

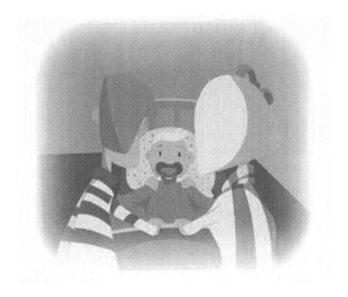

Why put an end to this wonderful thing called the pacifier? The (almost) only reason is that if the baby falls asleep with a pacifier, he or she will wake up at the end of every sleep cycle and will require it to be put back in his or her mouth.

And if not? The baby will not be able to transition into the next sleep cycle without it, and will be 100% dependent on it.

If your baby is addicted (a pacifier junkie, so to speak), now is the time to realize that the entire sleep process is dependent on the pacifier, and will continue to be until your child is 2-3-years old.

On the other hand, if your baby is a pacifier "refuser" – he or she must know why.

Twins Johnny and Kimberly were 6 months old when their parents decided that it was time for them to start sleeping at night. For 6 months, they breastfed, and when their mother began adding solid foods to their daily nutrition, she decided that it was time to teach them to sleep as well. Her neighbor Lisa, mother to a 4-month-old baby boy, enthusiastically shared with her that her son sleeps a full night, which also encouraged her to start teaching them to sleep.

She did not have a problem with the crying, because she said that they cried so much when they were tired that she felt that if they slept better, they would cry less during the day and night. Her problem was the pacifier. She had a hard time accepting that I ask they be weaned off of it, as it was the only thing that calmed them down.

I explained to Johnny and Kimberly's parents that during sleep, the pacifier falls out of their mouths anyway, and so there shouldn't be a problem asking them to not use a pacifier.

Regarding the pacifier's ability to "calm" the children, I explained that when babies at this age whine and are restless, it is usually because one of two things (Obviously this only relates to healthy babies):

Hunger – in which case they should not be given a pacifier but food (there are children who do not eat well because instead of food they are given a pacifier…I thought that this could be a great idea for a diet for me).

Tiredness – If the child is not hungry and is still whining and restless, then we can assume that he or she is tired and should be put to bed, rather than be given a pacifier to "calm down". The baby does not need to calm down, but to sleep.

On the first night the father "gave in" and gave Kimberly the pacifier after she had cried for 15 minutes, but the next night when they saw that Johnny had slept a full night and Kimberly still needed a pacifier for each sleep cycle, they threw away all the pacifiers.

They later called me with great joy to thank me and report that they had weaned both children off the pacifier forever!

Since this book deals with the overall welfare of babies and children, I encourage you parents to wean your children off the pacifier.

Let's admit it: The pacifier is for your benefit only. The baby cries – a pacifier is shoved in its mouth. Okay, well…not shoved, but put in its mouth. The baby nags – it's offered a pacifier. You're going somewhere in the car and you want a quiet ride, you give a pacifier. The baby is tired – you give a pacifier. Sometimes I see babies smiling with a pacifier in their mouth …as long as they are quiet. So here are a few facts before I explain why the method I developed for teaching babies to sleep does not include the use of a pacifier.

When a baby cries, one must first consider one of two main reasons for the crying: hunger or tiredness. If the child is hungry – he or she needs to be given food, not a pacifier. Sucking on a pacifier requires energy, which is a limited resource for babies, especially for those under 12 months old, and with diminished energy he will not eat as well (and if he doesn't eat well, he also won't sleep well).

If he or she is crying and isn't hungry, then the second reason to be considered is tiredness. If the baby is tired, he or she needs to sleep, a sleep which isn't dependent on any external object. If the baby falls asleep with the aid of a pacifier, it will need you to place it in its mouth every 90-120 minutes, between sleep cycles (at night), and every 20-45 minutes during the day. Whatever the baby falls asleep with when initially put down, is what he or she will require every sleep cycle.

With the method that I have developed, one of the main ideas is that the baby puts itself to sleep without any external objects, a pacifier or anything else. Without the dependency on an object, the baby can shift from one sleep cycle to the next independently. If the baby is tired, he or she needs to be put in bed without external aids. In the upcoming chapters I will teach you how to help your baby learn the skill of independently falling asleep. This will happen only when you will get rid of all the pacifiers you have at home. Yes, yes, right now—collect them, put them in box, make a note on it of the date on which you said goodbye to the pacifier, and keep it as a souvenir. Don't try to fool me by keeping one in your bag just in case… I see everything.

There are times when the baby wants a little touch, a hug. The pacifier is cold and detached, made of silicone, and it is most certainly no replacement for a hug or a touch. If you know that your baby is satiated and has slept enough, but is still nagging and seems unsatisfied – just pick him or her up and give hugs and kisses and smiles, and then another kiss. The pacifier is a (poor) replacement for touch. I have noticed that when babies nag and complain and not for hunger or tiredness, some parents will hurry to stick a pacifier in their mouth and quiet them down.

There is research evidence that using a pacifier in such cases may hinder the development of the baby's emotional intelligence. It happens by way of disabling the ability to express emotions by using facial mime, because they need to keep the pacifier in their mouth. The pacifier adversely affects the baby's ability to express emotions.

Sometimes I see a baby sitting in a stroller and observing his surroundings. Really wanting to talk or respond but…it has a pacifier in its mouth. To be a little less politically correct, I would say that the baby has a pacifier stuck in its mouth. I recommend leaving children's mouths open to be able to express everything they want to express, to develop their language and to enjoy their ever-developing language abilities. A pacifier hinders all of that.

The use of a pacifier over the age of 2-years-old could later cause issues in the structure of the bite, which is why the American Dental Association recommends weaning off the pacifier before the age of 2. To wean a child at the age of 2 (which is the adolescence of childhood) is a longer and more complicated process than not giving it to him or her to begin with, or to wean at a few months of age.

A pacifier is not a sterile object and there is always the possibility of contaminated elements sticking to it. Some of these disease sources that have been found in high prevalence include viruses, germs, and fungi. Contact of the pacifier rim with the lips, cheeks and chin, especially by a drooling child and for an extended period of time, encourages the development of skin infections and local inflammations. Not recommended!

Babies with pacifiers are at an increased risk (about twice as much) for contracting recurring inflammation of the middle ear.

I hope that I have managed to convince you to hang the pacifiers on the nearest pacifier tree in your neighborhood, and if you don't have one, you are invited to come over to my place – I have a fabulous pacifier tree.

I can further state that with the method I have developed it isn't possible to use a pacifier. The pacifier is a disruptive element for the child during the transitions between the sleep cycles, and will need it at every transition. Even if the child is already at the age where he or she can find the pacifier on his or her own (which happens at approximately 7 months) and put it in his or her mouth, he or she needs to wake up in order to do that – which itself disturbs sleep.

In cases where the parents put a few pacifiers around the child so he or she may find one more easily, the child stumbles upon them turning in bed, which also hinders good-quality sleep. So, if you want to utilize the method which I have developed to teach babies and children to put themselves to sleep and sleep all through the night, you will have to get rid of the pacifier. Even during the daytime because if the baby cries during the day, it means he or she is either hungry (and then needs to be fed), or tired, and even during the day needs to put him- or herself to sleep without the aid of external objects, because at night he or she will look for what he or she got during the day. And if the baby is crying for a hug or attention, then a silicone pacifier will never be a worthy replacement for a parental hug. Nothing is easier than to shove a pacifier in the baby's mouth to get it to be quiet, but that is not my philosophy as a mother or as a sleep coach. While night is only for sleep, during the day there needs to be hugging and playing, loving and admiration of the child's achievements; babies and children need to be met with enthusiasm. A pacifier cannot perform these functions.

In order to teach your baby how to sleep a full night, you first must take all the pacifiers out of the house. It's good for the sleeping process, it's excellent for dental reasons and it will allow you to avoid a significant weaning process which occurs around the age of 2 and up. So good-bye pacifier. Do not be afraid of this process. Just take it out of the house.

If the baby is under the age of 2, then they can be thrown away without the child seeing it. And if the child is already or almost 2 years old, what I suggest is to explain to him or her that now, at the age of 2, the pacifier is not healthy for teeth and mouth, and so it should end. You don't have to make a big deal out of it, or as the saying attributed to General Patton goes: **"If it won't be simple – It will simply not be!"**

When my son Itay weaned off pacifiers we waited early in the morning for the garbage truck (he was crazy about garbage trucks) and threw all of the pacifiers into the large truck dump. The sanitation workers applauded and smiled, but thinking back, it seems like a less educational thing to do. You don't throw things in the garbage, especially things which you have spent money on. But that's also an option… **Please Note:**

Despite the fact that the Department of Health supports giving breastfeeding babies a pacifier around the age of 4 weeks when the breastfeeding is already established, as a SIDS risk reducing factor, professional literature does not support this approach. The ultimate professional authority – the Cochrane Database Systemic Review, published a literature review on the subject. (Cochrane Database Syst Rev, 2017). The authors of the review summarize that there is no independent article that encourages or negates the use of a pacifier for the purpose of prevention of SIDS.

If you, the parents, want to give your baby a pacifier and he agrees to take it - you can give him the pacifier at bedtime and respond to him according to the method that is described in the book later in the night.

I realize how much contradicting indications confuse parents, and in the end it is you who will make the decisions what to do in accordance with your experience, knowledge as well as your baby's needs.

# Sleep...at the Mall

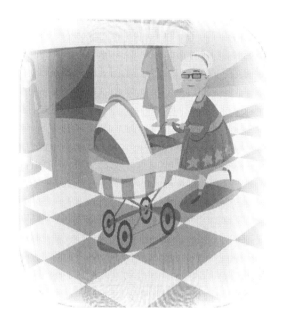

My grandmother always loudly professed that babies need to be taught to sleep anywhere. Even in daylight. She claimed babies need to be put to sleep during the day in a lit room, in the living room for example, and at night in a dark room.

What's amusing is that when she would go in for her sacred afternoon nap, she would go into her dark room and would not have anyone knock on her door or disturb her. I never saw her take a nap in the living room.

While it's true that sometimes there are situations when a child is tired and you cannot be at home in a dark room, if you are at home, he or she will fall asleep and sleep better in a dark room.

At the beginning of the skill-learning process I recommend being in the vicinity of the home for about a week (which is the length of time required to learn the sleeping skill with the "Shhh...at Night We Sleep" method). After a week of training, when the baby already knows how to put itself to sleep, it's okay to go out and have him or her fall asleep in all sorts of places outside the house. It's important to emphasize that outside the house the baby needs to be allowed to fall asleep using this method as well, and yet, you must take into consideration that the falling asleep process will take longer. Eventually... the baby will fall asleep, but will have a harder time than at home in a well-air-conditioned dark room. A baby is not a doll that immediately closes its eyes when you put it down. Parents who insist on having their baby fall asleep in the stroller at the shopping mall will need to pay the price, because he or she might cry and have difficulty falling asleep the next time that he or she needs to put himself to sleep.

**What can you do?**

First of all, start teaching the baby to put itself to sleep during the day and night in its room, in the dark, with a pleasant temperature of about 70-73 degrees (F). In the winter, closer to 73°F and in the summer more toward 70°F. After the sleeping process is established under these conditions, he or she can be taken out and you can let the falling-asleep process happen according to the method you choose. The important thing is to talk to the baby or child in the same manner and to act consistently, at home and away from home. Independent sleeping skills need to be established, and after that the baby will learn to fall asleep anywhere you go.

If you have plans to go shopping, for instance, I would recommend that you check on the baby before you want to leave the house. Is the baby rubbing its eyes or yawning? If the answer is yes, that means that this is the least appropriate time to go shopping, unless you have to, and then – as they say – you gotta do what you gotta do. If it's possible to leave the baby with a babysitter and go out alone – do that. During this time, your baby will sleep under the best conditions, assuring quality sleep.

If you have no one to leave the baby with, check if you have the option to delay the outing until after the baby sleeps. In this case the baby will sleep in a warm room in the winter or cool room in the summer, and when he or she wakes up he or she will be alert and happy, eat as much as necessary, and then you can take him or her shopping and the baby might even enjoy the sights, the sounds, and you. The right choice is to leave the house after the baby has awaken from a good, quality sleep and thus shopping can become a fun outing for both of you.

Sometimes we have wonderful plans and reality, let's admit it… gets in the way. If you need to leave the house and the baby is tired and you have no one to leave him or her with – it is advisable to be diligent about the guidelines of the method outside of the house as well. The most important thing is that the baby understands what is expected of him or her and understands that he or she needs to sleep now, even if he or she is not in his or her own bed. I promise you that after about three outings, if you act consistently and methodically, the baby will sleep well outside, too. Just remember: the process will take longer than it does at home and sometime may be accompanied by a greater frustration. Frustration is part of life, and this is a level of frustration which the baby can handle and even constitutes a part of its proper development. If you are the kind of parents who avoid putting the baby in frustrating situations as much as possible and you want to spare the child said frustration…don't go to the mall when the baby is tired. Always remember that the choice is yours.

There are parents who want to bring the baby along while running errands to strengthen their bond. While I agree that a joint outing (no matter where) may be a positive experience for both parties, if the baby is tired, there won't be a positive experience for either party. A tired, crying baby will cause you great frustration as parents, and fun for the baby is out of the question. If you decide to go to the mall with a tired baby, don't forget a large piece of cloth to cover the stroller. This way, with the relative darkness and the repetitive motions of the stroller, the baby might fall asleep. As long as this does not occur daily, it will not hinder the forming of any habit or method.

If you too have a grandmother who claims that the baby should know how to sleep in light and anywhere, then may I suggest that she take the baby to the shopping mall....

# Baby Wants – Baby Needs

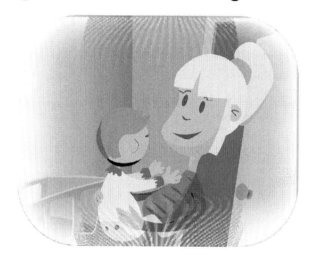

"He just wants to be held."

"She doesn't want to be in her car seat."

"She only wants to fall asleep in the stroller."

"He only agrees to eat if mommy feeds him." Guess what ages we're talking about here. Seven? Thirteen? No. These are sentences said by parents to babies who were just born.

A baby doesn't want; a baby just needs. When we talk about babies (under the age of 6 months), we need to understand that he or she still has not developed a will. Their world of concepts is exceptionally limited and it is the parents' responsibility to provide all of their needs. The parents must identify what the need is and provide it at the right time. In cases that you think the baby "wants" something, I would recommend to consider whether this is what your baby really needs. I recall one instance when a couple came to see me with a week-old baby because they were told that it's best to teach the baby how to sleep from birth before "bad habits" set in.

When they entered the clinic with a week-old, seven-pound baby, they told me that he cried the whole way because he doesn't like the car. I said to them, "Of course he doesn't, you have a Mazda, and maybe he would have preferred a BMW? You should have consulted him before purchasing the car."

They did not realize that a baby doesn't really grasp where he or she is placed. He cried because there was an unmet need. He was lacking in one of the two crucial physiological needs: food or sleep; he was either hungry or tired.

If the baby needs to eat, then he or she must be fed. If the baby needs to sleep, he or she must be put in bed to sleep. If the baby needs touch and caressing, he or she needs to be picked up, kissed, and hugged. It's always important to think in terms of what your baby needs. If a child needs all the food groups and doesn't need sugars, then keep everything but sugars in the house. If the baby wants cucumbers and doesn't want tomatoes – that's okay. In

that range, there is room for desires. It's important to note: this is age dependent. Starting at the age of 12 months, desires begin to develop. A baby can prefer a banana over strawberries, or can reach out towards objects he or she chooses, but the parents are still the ones who are required to keep identifying what it is that he or she needs, and provide him or her with them.

When it comes to a want, parents may indulge that want within the guidelines of reason. This is part of the respect that a child deserves. Having said that, when the child needs to sleep there is no room to question. For example, whether he or she wants to go to bed or prefers to sleep with his parents. This isn't an option, unless your outlook on life is that the right thing is to have communal family sleeping or that the child needs to be given everything it wants, in which case this book might not be for you. The approach in this book is of respect for the baby and child by fulfilling both their physical and emotional needs, while including boundaries for safety.

So when your baby or child is crying, think for a moment what the need is—what he or she needs now. If the baby needs touch, give touch, don't stick a pacifier in its mouth. If the baby is hungry, feed it as much as he or she needs—no less, no more. If he or she is tired, he or she needs to get into bed to sleep and fall asleep on his or her own. There is no such thing as a baby who doesn't like its bed. He or she doesn't need to like it, but rather needs to get in it and sleep. This is the baby's task. In the upcoming chapters you will learn how to be your baby's guides, because this is all that he or she needs: for you to teach him or her how to sleep independently.

*Did you know?*

*Abraham Maslow defined the Hierarchy of Needs according to the order of importance. After having fulfilled the biological needs, a person is able to fill the other needs. Sleep is a basic physiological need.*

**Self Fulfillment:**
morality, creativity,
spontaneity, problem solving,
lacking prejudice, accepting reality

**Respect & Admiration:**
self esteem, confidence, success,
respecting others, respected by others

**Sense of Belonging, Identity, and Love:**
friendship, family, sexual intimacy

**Physical Assurance:**
of the body, work, resources, morality, family, health, belongings

**Basic Physiology Needs:**
oxygen, food, water, sleep, homeostasis, relieving

# Food, a Bath, and to Bed

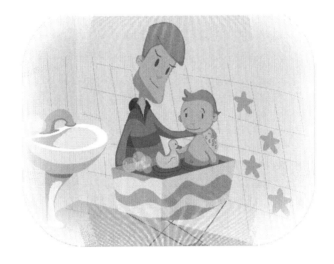

Before the process of putting a baby to sleep at night begins, there are a few important actions which need to be performed with the baby, namely, supper and a bath.

I know what you're thinking: First dinner and only then a bath? The answer is yes, and you will soon understand why. But first, let us speak of routines. A routine is a set of actions in a consistent order. There is nothing like a routine for babies and children, and honestly, it's also great for us adults. It creates order, provides a sense of security, and it's essential to one's peace of mind.

With the "Shhh…at Night We Sleep" method, the routine starts with supper preceding the bath. I love that babies get into the bath when they are well-fed. That way, they are calmer in the bath and the messes made while eating are cleaned off the baby. There are parents who choose not to bathe their child every day for different reasons and that's fine. It's possible to bathe the baby as needed and there is no need to make that an inseparable part of the method's routine.

## Food

The amount of calories which a baby or child requires for growth needs to be consumed during the day. Babies who will not eat during the night should eat more during the day so that the amount of calories that they consume will be kept constant. During the day, babies need to eat approximately five times. The question of "how much" is irrelevant when healthy babies who came to term are concerned. A baby (and a child) needs to eat when he or she wants to and as much as he or she wants to (as long as it isn't during the times he or she is supposed to sleep). Each baby and child has its own metabolism and I object to tables which indicate how much the baby has to eat. Trust your baby to eat as much as he or she needs. If you are worried about his or her health or weight, you can always consult a doctor or a child-development nurse, but in general the amount of calories a baby consumes depends on various factors: the weather or ambient temperature, body movements, the amount of energy expended that day, genetics, and more. It is very important to know that during the first year of life fat cells are formed, which is why the baby's nourishment during the first year is so important and critical to the health of the person which he or she will grow up to be. Later in life, fat cells may shrink or expand, but their number will remain constant throughout life. Babies and children who have eaten more than they wanted (because their parents insisted on "just another bite") are babies who may become members of a group with risk factors for future obesity. This is why I recommend coming to supper with the children in a quiet and calm frame of mind, and not worry about how much he or she will eat. Leave those worries to grandma.

Regarding **supper**, I would like to emphasize a few principles:

Supper should be eaten in the kitchen or the dining area –food is to be eaten in the location intended for it. There are parents of children ages 5 and up that go crazy because their child is unable to sit quietly at the table and will only eat in the living room. The reason for this behavior is that when he or she was a baby that is where they were fed. When the child grew up and the parents decided to change his or her habits, the child resisted, and rightfully so! If your family is in the habit of eating in the living room and you expect it to continue that way, then this paragraph isn't for you.

The baby needs to eat as much as he or she wants. Even if during the night he or she will not be eating, the baby does not have to eat a lot in the evening. On the contrary –

The less he or she eats at dinner, the better he or she will sleep. With the "Shhh…at Night We Sleep" method you eat in accordance with the 12th century Jewish philosopher Maimonides' instructions: in the morning you eat like a king, at lunchtime like a prince and in the evening like a pauper. Just don't put the child on a diet. If he or she wants to eat a lot – well, good for them! If he or she eats a little – well, also good for them. For babies who already eat solids I recommend that dinner be comprised more of the solids and less of milk. The more solids and less fluids in the meal, the better and longer the sleep. If you don't want to give up the bottle of formula, you can offer the baby the bottle right after eating solids. If you are breastfeeding then, obviously, you can breastfeed after the meal, as long as it is in the well-lit dining area and the baby doesn't fall asleep on the breast. Breastfeeding and falling asleep need to be detached.

Avoid giving cereals of sorts. It is an unnecessary load on the digestive system. Cereals are good in the morning, when the digestive system is at its best, not so at night.

A family meal is very important and the desirable situation is for the entire family to sit around the table together for the evening meal. Children are very observant and tend to imitate their parents' eating and drinking habits.

The family meal is an excellent opportunity to watch the parents eat all of the foods that should be on the table in terms of the food groups. A child who observes his parents eating a variety of foods in a polite manner will do the same, I promise you! The process may take months. Be patient, and you will see that one day the child will reach out for something that you thought he or she would never touch. While we are on the subject of family dinners, I would like to mention an issue which isn't directly linked to the method: many parents don't take their eyes off their children's plates, and that is a mistake. Beyond the fact that this may cause an eating disorder, it is impolite and at certain ages can cause the child not to eat what the parents want him or her to (out of spite). The right thing to do is have every member of the family around the table mind their own plate. Starting as early as 12 months it's possible (and recommended) to wait for the baby to point at what he or she wants and to allow him or her to eat as much as he or she wants and prefers. It's possible of course to offer food, but first wait for the child to express a desire, and if that doesn't happen then offer food only once.

It's important the child not eat too much but only what he or she needs, and even if that isn't a lot, that's okay—he or she will actually sleep better. Pressure will not increase the child's desire to eat, just the opposite. I wouldn't put a child on a diet, of course, but just remember it's important that he or she eats enough during the day.

I may have shattered a few myths for some mothers, but lay off the pressure about food. The age of running after your child with "one last bite" is over. Trust your children that if they are hungry, they will eat. Many parents don't give their children a chance to even ask for food, they just keep offering and offering. Stop doing that. It's their responsibility, and if you don't agree with me that your child will know how to signal when he or she is hungry or to explicitly ask for food, then offer it, but only once. Don't nag children about food.

Another important thing to remember about babies and children: the stomach is not a particularly large muscle, despite its tendency to expand. It is ill-advised to overload it with more food than the baby needs. Babies and children need to eat just enough. It may seem to us as parents that the amount is too small, but babies and children know how much they need. They know how to signal to us not only when they are hungry, but also when they are full. Listen to them. At any age. When the baby has already progressed to solids (at 4-6 months) it's advisable to try a new vegetable or fruit every day and note the re-actions. Was he relaxed? Did she develop a rash? How well did he sleep that day? When babies eat solids they can sleep for a longer period of time. The more babies eat solids and fats (healthy fats, unsaturated fats) the longer the food stays in the stomach and that has a positive impact on their sleep.

It is important to emphasize that at these ages solid food is not a substitute for breastfeeding or formula. If you wish to continue breast-feeding (and I strongly recommend it), you can continue while you combine small meals of solid food, which will also expose the baby to new tastes and textures.

Some parents tell me that their baby has not gained weight and that they are stressed about it. To push food into a child's mouth is not the solution, instead, let him or her reach a state of hunger, and then offer food. Babies are very smart creatures and will quickly realize if they are dealing with parents who constantly want to fuss with food, and then they will resist. Yes, almost at any age. One exception: with especially small babies or preemies, doctors' orders must be followed.

One more thing: during the family dinner I recommend putting the cell phones on silent. No phone conversations during dinner! Remember the golden rule about how children watch and learn what and how to eat. You are their role model. When they grow up it will be difficult for you to ask them to put their phones aside during supper. They will remember all too well that you did not practice what you are preaching. You will not need to wait long before they get to the age where they mimic you and want to have their meal with their iPad next to them. Behave today as you would want them to behave in the future. There are parents who tell me that they like to allow their children to play with their iPad when they eat out because then they get some quiet time and the children can sit for longer at the table. I think that's wonderful. If that suits you too, you can do that.

Now, for the issue troubling many parents: what is the right time to teach a baby to stop eating at night?

The answer is clear. Babies who were brought to term, weigh six-and-a-half pounds or more, and are considered healthy babies, may skip night feeding and sleep through the night when they're 3-months-old. It's fine if you decide to wait they're 4-months-old. Some pediatricians recommend teaching the baby how to sleep a full night even before the age of 3 months if the baby weighs at least 11 pounds. Sounds like a fantasy? Then you should know that this could be your reality. If your baby was born on time, is now at least 3-months- old, weighs over 11 pounds and is a healthy baby, according to my system he or she will sleep a full night of 10-12 hours nonstop and learn how to do so, on average, within three days. In the case of preemies or babies who weigh less, they should be fed during the night until 4-5 (adjusted age), and only then allowed to relinquish this meal. If you have a baby who was born prematurely and don't know his or her adjusted age, I recommend consulting a pediatrician or a sleep coach to help with the calculation.

Sleep is critical for two important systems: The part of the brain called the Hippocampus (responsible for, among other things, learning and memory processes that occur during sleep), and the immune system. Sleep is important for the regulation of the biological clock. Internal and external sleep interruptions interfere with the biological clock and weaken the immune system significantly.

Babies need to **sleep at night**, not eat. Calorie intake will be made up for during the day. Babies who sleep well at night follow their growth chart better because during uninterrupted sleep the pituitary gland secretes the growth hormone which, as suggested in its name, assists in the baby's growth processes. A baby doesn't grow with food. Grandmothers always say that babies grow in their sleep, and they're right!

There are parents who swear that because their baby drinks an entire bottle, "it's not possible that he's not hungry." I'm here to tell you, dear parents, that the baby isn't hungry, but has simply developed the habit of eating at night. Babies are fond of habits and they acquire them very quickly. It's not just babies who develop habits this quickly: if you wake me up at three o'clock in the morning and give me my favorite snack I, too, will wake up every night at 3 AM to look for it, and my stomach will yearn for it. That is the force of habit.

> **Did you know?**
>
> *There is nothing stronger than the force of habit!*

During the first three months of its life a baby must eat at night because the stomach at this stage is small, fills with milk only and empties quickly. Even when the stomach grows the baby continues to wake up at the same hours because it has gotten used to being fed…at night.

It is the parents' role to realize that this routine was appropriate at a certain age, but one day you need to stop this habit and say: "That's it, from now on my baby doesn't need to eat at night, he needs to sleep." If three months seems too early to you, you can extend it to four to five months. Even six months is reasonable, but beyond that you should know that sleep disturbances and sleep deprivation cause health issues. In the upcoming chapters I will talk about changing this habit. From the day you become aware of this important information, your capability to look after your baby's health grows. This book will support you in the process. A noble cause is before you: to teach your babies and children the skill of falling asleep on their own and sleeping through the entire night.

**A breastfeeding baby:** if your baby is only breastfeeding, especially if your baby is not yet at an age where he or she is eating solids, it is important to breastfeed upon demand. A baby breastfeeds when it wants and as much as it wants. It is important to make sure that the baby does not fall asleep on the breast. If you notice that his or her eyes are shutting, stop breastfeeding for a moment, and offer to finish the meal on the other breast, just as long as he or she doesn't fall asleep while suckling. If the baby falls asleep while feeding, the brain remembers! During the process of going to sleep and in between sleep cycles he or she will wait for the nipple as well as the sensation of the food going into the stomach (especially at a time when he or she doesn't need this food). If your baby is only breastfeeding I suggest that just before you put him or her to bed that you offer an additional session only to make sure that he or she is satiated. If he or she isn't hungry, then he or she will immediately push out the breast nipple (I call it the breast-test). A baby who isn't hungry will not keep eating.

**When the baby is on formula:** If your baby is fed formula, you should feed him or her according to need. If he or she is a healthy baby, you need to add 1/3 oz. every day until the bottle is full. Don't worry about loading the child with too much food. Babies know how to push the nipple or the bottle away when they are full. We adults have lost our biological awareness for feeling hunger and satiation (at least some of us). This mechanism still works fabulously in babies. If the baby ate a little more than he or she needed to, then he or she will spit up the surplus. Don't worry when this occurs, unless it happens often and then you should consult a pediatrician.

## Bath

Bath time is not just for body cleaning, it's also the parents' quality time with their baby. Parents smile at the thought of bath time with the baby. Both parties have fun. The parents especially enjoy seeing their baby smile and delighted during this quality time. Water always reminds babies of the pleasant stay in the womb, the touch of the baby's skin by the parents is always pleasant, and that makes this time really fun. I think that parents need this "together time" the most. They may be away from the house most hours of the day and view it as a way to make up for the time they didn't spend with the baby during the day. I'm sure that many of you parents agree with me. Even if you have been with the baby the entire day, bath time is a time to pleasantly bring the day's joint activities to an end.

I don't want to be a party pooper, but remember that "life is like a grocery store, you have to pay for everything in the end."

The "price" of the fun for the baby will be difficulty in parting with this quality time, and the "price" for the parents is the heartache caused by the baby's hardship. What baby would want to part with the parents after such a fun bath time, especially since the levels of adrenaline (the arousal hormone) rise as a result of the playing, singing, and mutual smiles that accompany bath time?

I used to love bathing my children every night before going to bed. It felt right in terms of hygiene habits, the mutual pleasure derived from it, as well as part of the sleep ritual. Some say parents should bathe the baby twice a week or as needed. There are those who claim that over-bathing (daily) is not good because it could remove the natural skin oils. This approach is more and more prevalent today and you can adopt it if it suits you. Parents know and feel when a baby needs a bath. The frequency of bathing is your decision and is not directly linked to the method. So whether you like to bathe the baby daily like me, or less often, when you do bathe the baby remember a few things: Be prepared! Some of the things that I will ask you to do as part of the "Shhh…at Night We Sleep" method may not be to your liking, but I am convinced that after you read the explanation, you might accept these guidelines, if not with love, then with understanding.

The bath needs to be taken following supper. At any age. Babies who suffer from reflux of the digestive system need to have their bath prior to the meal. (This is a normal occurrence in babies and can turn into a digestive disruption. It manifests itself in flow of food or fluids in the opposite direction – from the stomach back up the esophagus. It is a phenomenon that can occur at any age, but is most common in babies and is the number one cause of spitting up and throwing up in infancy. The peak of this phenomenon is around the age of 4 months. Reflux usually ends on its own, especially when it occurs in babies.) Except for this specific case, all other babies and children should take a bath after the meal when they are satiated and relaxed. It's advisable to make sure that you put a baby before the age of 3 months on a bouncer or in your arms for about 5-10 minutes after the meal before putting him or her in the bath. Let them rest for a few minutes after the meal (just make sure that he or she doesn't start to fall asleep). When you put the baby in the bath, make sure you don't flip him or her around; after all, he or she did just have a meal. It's possible to clean the baby thoroughly with minimum movements. The reason why children should be put in the bath after the meal and not before is that after the meal, when babies and children are full, they can better enjoy bath time. A hungry baby might cry a lot during bath time, which is an unpleasant experience for both parties. Some children also spit up after they eat and some get dirty with food. Why not eat first and then bathe and get into bed all clean? I also think that many children do not like to take a bath when they grow up because they remember bath time as an unpleasant experience, and I think the origin of this is a distant memory of being in the water while hungry. My clinical experience is that babies seem happier and calmer during bath time when they have already eaten.

*Now, here are two important rules concerning the bath before bed time:*

Bath time should not exceed two minutes - maximum. Don't look surprised. The rationale behind this instruction is that babies and children have a hard time with transitions. If they have too much fun in the bath with toys and songs it will be difficult for them to part with all the fun, and the process of getting into bed in a dark room will be harder. We want to make things easier on our babies and children. We want to lower the adrenaline levels during the transition between the fun active day and the quiet dark night. The more fun and stimulating the bathing is, the more difficult it will be to go to sleep. On the other hand, I would not want babies and children to give up on the bath time fun. They really love it, and baths are part of pleasant childhood memories. I suggest a weekend "Fun Bath" of unlimited duration, with toys, accompanied by songs and joy. The children will really wait for this special time. There is another option, which is to have this bath everyday right after coming home from daycare. That is a period of time long enough before bedtime, and then you can have the bath with all the fun, toys and joy. This will be early enough not to effect going to sleep at the end of the day.

During bath time it's best to have only one parent present in the bathroom (unless you have twins). Why is that so important? For two reasons:

When both parents are in the bathroom, parting with both of them afterwards is more difficult for the baby. It's easier for the baby to say good-bye to one parent when going to bed.

With children it's always best to think ahead. One of the problems of first-born children is that when they are still an only child, both parents will be with him or her in the bathroom (as well as at other times). When a year or more passes and a new baby is added to the family, all of a sudden only one parent is present, and that is linked directly to the notion that the new baby has taken a parent away from the older child. Issues of jealousy may arise, accompanied by a variety of regressions related to the new addition to the family. If the baby is used to having only one parent bathe him, then when additional siblings arrive it will already be natural to have only one of the parents bathing, and thus one of the most difficult issues of the arrival of a new baby can be avoided.

Everything that we do according to this system is to make things easier for your baby and child. There's a reason they say "God is in the details." There is an importance to (almost) everything. These guidelines are for the welfare of the baby and child and the meeting of his or her physiological and emotional needs.

*Let's summarize the bath topic:*

**For babies 3-18 months-old:**
A short (1-2 minute) bath, no special stimulus, one toy maximum, no singing or playing. If the baby talks and makes sounds, he or she shouldn't be silenced, of course, but should be responded to quietly (and don't forget the smile).

**For older children:**

If the child wants to stay in the bath longer, you quietly explain that there is a longer bath time waiting on the weekend. Promise a "Fun Bath" on Saturday or Sunday, and he or she will have something to look forward to. If the child asks why bath time is short and with no games, explain what you've learned (which is that it will make going to sleep easier… that when we take a bath that is filled with toys and fun we create in our body something [a hormone] which makes it harder to fall asleep.) This explanation should be age appropriate, of course. If the child asks for "just one more minute," allow it.

An additional minute with older children will not cause any drama. Entering into a power struggle over this would be a huge mistake. There is a risk that the child will then ask for "one more last minute" and this is where you explain (calmly) that agreements need to be honored. He or she asked for another minute and you allowed it, and now he or she too needs to be considerate of the parents' needs. It would be a good idea to say: "I need to take a shower too, to end the day and get ready for bed, and I trust you to understand that and respect what I ask of you." This kind of a dialogue is respectful to both parties. Remember: You do not need to be tough with children. You just need to be determined and most importantly - consistent. In the mobile phone age, it's best to program an alarm after one or two minutes. This helps children with boundaries.

There are parents who claim that the bath is what makes the child tired, and they think that he or she sleeps better that way. If this is the case for you and you don't have an issue with the baby or child's parting, and the going-to-sleep process is calm and pleasant, then by all means keep on the practice of a funfilled bath that the child is used to. Don't change a winning team.

As a rule, this is a good time to mention that whatever works for you doesn't need to be replaced by another action. Pick what's right and suits you. Whatever works differently is wonderful. Stick with it.

After food and bath, it's time for:

## Bed

There are parents who allow their children to go back to the living room after food and bath for games or even a story or two. Parents have told me that they read an entire library because the child wants another book, and another, and another, and one last one, and then just one more, and play with Lulu the Bear… So let's talk about this issue for a moment.

Reading books (at any age) is fabulous. A story contains all the elements required for development: vocabulary, imagination, quality time, reading habits, focusing, and more. All of these wonderful things which reading books does for children need to be done during the day, not before bedtime, which is when we want to lower the adrenaline levels (the arousal hormone). Bedtime stories can manifest themselves in unwanted dreams, not to mention scary dreams. Our subconscious has a field day with these bedtime stories (as may also happen with stories that are told during the day), but the likelihood of a flower in a story turning into a monster in a dream is higher when the story is told at bedtime. Bedtime is not for doing things that should have been done during the day. Bedtime is a time to take leave of the day's activities and shift down gears, not to start a new parent-child experience. Children have a hard time parting with their parents for the night, so they ask for another story and another and another and just one more. They are less interested in the story itself and more focused on not parting with the parent. But sleep is no less important! Parents should be aware of this and invest this quality time during the day. When a parent comes home only in the evening, this quality time will wait for the weekend.

This is not such a bad thing. It's better to have quality time once or twice a week and good sleeping habits throughout the week. The baby or child does not need to suffer because the parent returns home from work only at 7 or 8 PM. The parent shouldn't feel bad, all they were doing is going out to make a living. On a personal note, my entire life I was a mother and a provider. It's my experience that it's possible to make a living working nine to five. It doesn't always require coming home at 8 PM (obviously there are jobs which require unconventional hours and one can (and should) make an effort to come home a few days a week at hours when you and your child can enjoy each other). It's all a matter of cost and gain, and mostly of choices.

When a baby or child gets into bed after stories, games and fun, he or she is full of adrenaline and will have a hard time transitioning into the falling asleep stage in this hormonal condition. As I write these lines I recall the times that I would come home after delivering babies on an evening shift. The adrenaline surge that I would have after such an amazing childbirth experience would really get in the way of my falling asleep. The same happens with babies and children. While they did not just return from the delivery room, they have just finished sharing time with their parent, playing, laughing, and the adrenaline might get in the way of their falling asleep. So if we want to help the baby in the process, we need to do this: around 6 PM we should shift down gears, lower the level of activity, start picking up toys, turn off the TV, stop singing, and refrain from introducing any special fun. Quality time and fun should end by 6 PM at the latest. Most babies and children need to **sleep** by around 7 PM. Until what age? Five!

At age 6, you can push it back by about half an hour to an hour. Of course, if you have any personal restrictions, arrange the time according to your needs, but I believe the idea is clear. Just know that children need about 10-12 hours of nonstop sleep, while adults need less, about 8 (more or less). Babies and children are in a growth process which requires a lot of energy and they need many more hours of sleep then we adults do.

If your babies and children still show signs of difficulty parting with you, that's okay. This hardship needs to be understood and even taken as a big compliment. They have had fun with you during the day or during the hours prior to sleep. The fact that they are having a hard time getting into bed is natural, and absolutely normal. It's important that you as parents don't show pity and take them out of bed or get them used to falling asleep only in your presence. This is where boundaries must be set for you (not the children).

If you stay with the baby or child, you will be making two kinds of mistakes:

You are sending a message that he or she cannot stay alone and manage the sleep process on his or her own.

You - how can I put this gently? - are sort of cheating your child. Your child will shut his eyes when you are next to him, but when he opens his eyes between sleep cycles you will no longer be there. This is, by the way, how anxieties can develop. Mom was here and all of a sudden she disappeared. It's very important the baby or child understand the falling asleep process is his and his alone. If you have been good parents all day, providing your children with everything that they need physically and emotionally, putting them down and expecting them to put themselves to sleep is a completely realistic expectation, it relays the message "Yes you can". It goes without saying that I believe parents deserve to sleep as well. The fact that you had a baby doesn't mean that your basic rights have been revoked. At night, everyone sleeps (except for owls, bats, and other nocturnal creatures). Humans are active during the day and sleep at night. Historically, people would turn in at sunset and wake up at dawn. Ever since Thomas Edison invented the light bulb in 1879 people started going to sleep later and changed their biological clock. Babies and children still sleep during hours which are closer to sunset and sunrise, which is why many parents aren't happy (to say the least) when their children wake up around 5:00-5:30AM. From the children's point of view, they went to sleep around 6:30PM and woke up at sunrise, but the parents stayed up to watch TV, went out with friends or to a show and had a hard time waking up early the next morning with the children. I have two (not ideal) solutions:

During the week try to go to bed as early as possible. Go out on the weekend. My husband and I, for example, decided that Friday evenings are dedicated to going out. During the rest of the week we went to bed at a time which will allowed us a good 8-9 hours of sleep.

When the baby wakes at 5:30AM, say good morning, turn on the light, give him or her breakfast, turn off the light, and go back to sleep. You would be surprised how many of them will go back to sleep even for another hour and a half or two. Some won't want to go back to sleep after having started the morning. That's okay too, especially if they slept all through the night.

If these two solutions are not feasible as far as you're concerned, know that this stage too shall pass. Children grow up and the time comes when you can go back to sleep as much as you like. I am currently at that stage and it's wonderful. Middle age is something to look forward to.

I hope I've convinced you that you (and your children) deserve to sleep. Sleep, sleep, **just sleep**.

I am all for including the children (at any age!) in on this idea. The baby also can (and should) be taught that **mom and dad need their sleep, too.** The child needs to grow with social awareness of the need to be considerate of others. They're not alone in this world. This will help them become better, happier people. Research shows that a child raised to possess social awareness and the ability to be considerate of others will have a greater sense of value, which will increase his or her sense of happiness. I believe that this is an ability that needs to be developed from infancy. It's okay to say to the baby: You got food (as much as you needed), you received a thousand kisses, play time, you are bathed and clean, you are a beloved baby, special and cherished, and now **we all need to sleep**. We, the parents, as well.

One of my fondest memories from bedtime as a little girl is the lullaby which my mother sang to me. Sometimes my dad would put us to sleep and then he would recite a different poem. There was "mom's lullaby" or "dad's poem," depending on whose responsibility it was to put me to bed.

That's why when parents ask me if it's okay to sing a lullaby to the baby or child when he or she is put down, I say: "Absolutely!" My mother used to sing me a lullaby of two verses (only while writing this book I discovered that it actually has more). At that moment, it occurred to me that she already wanted to end her day and that is why she cut it short. I am convinced that had I known as a child that there were more verses I would have insisted that she sing the whole song to me.

> *Hush, little baby, don't say a word.*
> *Papa's gonna buy you a mockingbird*
> *And if that mockingbird won't sing,*
> *Papa's gonna buy you a diamond ring*
> *And if that diamond ring turns brass,*
> *Papa's gonna buy you a looking glass*
> *And if that looking glass gets broke,*
> *Papa's gonna buy you a billy goat*
> *And if that billy goat won't pull,*
> *Papa's gonna buy you a cart and bull*
> *And if that cart and bull turn over,*
> *Papa's gonna buy you a dog named Rover*

*And if that dog named Rover won't bark*
*Papa's gonna buy you a horse and cart*
*And if that horse and cart fall down,*
*You'll still be the sweetest little baby in town.*

If my father would return before I would fall asleep, he would come to my bed and wrap me up in my blanket "like a fish" – as he put it – and recite a wonderful poem by Laura Richards:

*Goodnight, Sun! Go to bed!*
*Take your crown from your shining head.*
*Now put on your gray nightcap,*
*And shut your eyes for a good long nap.*
*Goodnight, Sky, bright and blue!*
*Not a wink of sleep for you.*
*You must watch us all the night,*
*With your twinkling eyes so bright.*
*Goodnight, flowers! Now close up Every swinging bell and cup.*
*Take your sleeping-draught of dew:*
*Pleasant dreams to all of you!*
*Goodnight, birds, that sweetly sing!*
*Little head 'neath little wing!*
*Every leaf upon the tree*
*Soft shall sing your lullaby.*
*Last to you, little child,*
*Sleep is coming soft and mild.*
*Now sleep shuts your blue eyes bright:*
*Little child dear, goodnight!*

My father would recite all the verses of the poem and then give me a kiss and at that moment it was clear that I had to go to sleep. That is how they would do it with all five of us. There was love, there was attention, and there were very clear boundaries. I thank my parents for that. This did not leave us an inch to start asking for food or drink and another story and another.

We received all the attention and love during the day, but at night there was a clear-cut message: **"It's night time…and we sleep!"**

My parents always told people with a smile that at 8 PM they were their "own masters," and maybe that was one of their secrets to a wonderful partnership that lasted 45 years until my father passed away. They always had the evening to themselves despite the fact that they raised five children, which they had within just eight years.

> *Did you know?*
>
> *Consistency is the key and the basis to any system you choose.*

# Breastfeeding or Formula – It's Not a Question!

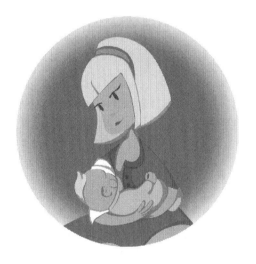

Breastfeeding or formula is not even a question.

Breastfeeding is one of the topics on which there is full consensus. It's not a matter of opinion, it's a fact: breastfeeding is the healthiest way to feed your baby.

The ingredients, the temperature, the flow of the milk from the nipple – all of these make mother's milk the superfood for your baby. It's extremely rare a baby has sensitivity to its mother's breast milk. On the other hand, many babies have all sorts of reactions to different formulas available on the market.

The advantages of breastfeeding are important and varied for both mother and child.

## Advantages for the baby

Breast milk is clean, germ free, and contains anti-inflammatory components.

Breast milk contains many enzymes which play an important role in the health and development of the baby. It contains enzymes which help the baby digest the milk sugars, fats, different carbs, and promote calcium absorption.

Statistically, breastfed babies have fewer infections, inflammations, and other diseases. Breast milk contains anti-infection elements which eliminate germs and other infectious elements in the digestive system. For example, the lactoferrin in breast milk operates with other antigens to suppress the development of E.coli, which is the most common reason for digestive contaminations in babies.

Breast milk contains antibodies against a variety of illnesses that the mother was exposed to. When the baby breastfeeds he or she is immediately exposed to a variety of organisms which the mother has already been exposed to.

Breast milk contains lactoferrin, a protein which acts as a binding agent for iron, and assists in its absorption.

Breastfeeding babies develop fewer chronic and autoimmune diseases during their lives, such as Crohn's, early onset diabetes, childhood arthritis, and multiple sclerosis.

Breastfeeding babies suffer from fewer allergies. Breast milk assists in the maturing of the digestive system and creates a protective lining in the intestines, thus decreasing the instances of allergies.

Breast milk contains elements suitable to the baby's age, thus it is the most appropriate for preemies whose digestive system has not matured and might have difficulties digesting food. Breast milk is the easiest to digest, is the most suitable to their special needs, and gives them the highest level of protection from diseases. Preemies nourished with breast milk develop better neurologically than those feeding on formula.

Breastfeeding doesn't just provide nourishment. It strengthens the emotional bond between mother and child. Mothers report with great pleasure the enormous feeling of satisfaction at producing the (healthiest and best) food for their baby. It's no wonder that there are women who have a really hard time weaning off breastfeeding even when their baby is ready for it.

## Advantages for the mother

During the first few days after labor, breastfeeding assists in the contracting of the uterus, decreases bleeding, and promotes weight loss.

Breastfeeding decreases the chances of breast cancer and ovarian cancer.

Breastfeeding decreases loss of calcium and thus decreases the risk for osteoporosis later in life.

Breast milk is always clean and ready to eat. It does not require any preparation and is available on demand at the exact right temperature at all hours of the day and night. It eliminates the need for bottles, washing, cleaning and sterilization of the equipment.

Breastfeeding is free, saving money on formulas and bottles which are rather costly.

Breastfeeding delays a woman's return to fertility, a benefit for those who do not wish to get pregnant so soon after the birth of the baby. It is important to remember, however, that it isn't a foolproof contraceptive.

You might be surprised, but breastfeeding has disadvantages as well:

Breastfeeding requires energy, and infants are still tired and unable to suckle efficiently, which may at times inhibit the production of breast milk. This may cause prolonged nursing which is very tiresome to both mother and baby.

It isn't possible to measure the amount of food that the baby has. Many times a baby will nurse a little and stop when still not satiated and then have a hard time falling asleep, and the mother will not know what the reason for the difficulty is because she has already breastfed. With a bottle it is clear to see if the baby had an amount which seems sufficient.

Only the mother can provide breast milk and she is unable to be assisted by a family member even following a difficult delivery or during an illness.

After breastfeeding for a prolonged period the baby might have difficulty transitioning to a bottle.

Breastfeeding may have complications. These are not a normal part of breastfeeding, but should be noted: breast congestion, nipple sores, breast mastitis and more.

There are women whose breast shape changes following breastfeeding.

## Formula

There are cases in which the mother is not allowed to breastfeed, usually for medical reasons, and then the baby formula is an excellent substitute. Sometimes it's the parents' choice, and it is theirs to make.

As opposed to the recommendation to choose one formula and stick with it, I recommend changing formulas every time you finish a container. Past experience has shown that certain formulas may lack a certain component crucial for the growth and development of babies, and thus caution should be exercised until the time that the baby starts eating solids.

Health is a wide concept and depends on how the entire life is conducted and not just infancy. So if a mother is forced or chooses to feed her baby formula, she is in no way a bad mother, and her children can be healthy and happy just like all breastfeeding babies. It really depends on things in years to come.

The mother-child bond doesn't depend on breastfeeding. Parents who fed their baby formula can create a wonderful bond with their baby. The parent-child bond is not dependent on the breast alone. The parent-child bond is comprised of so many factors, dear mother, you shouldn't feel uncomfortable or worry about your bond with your child if you cannot or don't want to breastfeed. The bond created while feeding can be developed with a bottle as well.

When you nurse the baby with formula you should make sure of a few things:

When you feed the baby, keep eye contact. This is how he or she learns to link you to the good food he or she is receiving.

During feeding, I recommend not talking on the phone. Concentrate on the feeding action only. This is a time which is important for both you and the baby.

If by any chance you are combining breastfeeding and formula, or breast milk in a bottle, make sure you use a bottle with a nipple that imitates the size of the opening in your nipple. Too large, and the baby will not want to go back to the breast. In a nipple with big openings the food comes out easier and the baby will always look for the easiest way to get food.

And on a personal note...to parents using baby formula:

Despite the fact that I am a great advocate of breastfeeding, and as far as I am concerned it is the best way to nourish your baby, I am a big believer that mothers know what is right for them and their baby. Breastfeeding is not the only measure of good motherhood. It is a (small) part of it. Your mental health and your state of mind are more important than the kind of milk that you nourish your child with. When my children were born – I have three – I knew how important breastfeeding was. I made great efforts to breastfeed. It wasn't easy for me. My nipples got sores from day one. I was never confident that the milk was enough. Every cry was accompanied by a great doubt that they may be hungry. On my first visit to the child-development clinic with my eldest, Shir, when the scale showed no increase in weight, I literally broke down. I cried my eyes out. I felt like a failure. I felt that I couldn't count on myself, that I was not a good mother. I immediately stopped breastfeeding. The quiet and sound sleep which followed the bottle of formula reinforced my confidence that I was doing the right thing. That story pretty much repeated itself with my next son and my daughter. I breastfed them all… until I observed that they were restless and not gaining weight. Then, like a cheerleading group in a basketball game, my sisters, my parents, and my husband begged me to give up breastfeeding and move on to a bottle.

Being a breastfeeding coach, I too, am an advocate of this priceless liquid called breast milk, but I remind all those women who can't (or don't want to) breastfeed that it's okay. Not perfect, but most certainly okay. Breast milk is good for all babies, but not for all mothers, and mothers also need to put themselves in a place that is good for them. In that same way, the "Shhh… at Night We Sleep" method is suitable for all the babies in the world, but it isn't suitable for all mothers (and fathers). That is okay too. Make a decision that you can live with in peace and happiness. You, the parents, will make many decisions regarding the raising of your children and their education in the marathon of life. These decisions will not always be ideal but remember that "the greatest enemy of the good is…the best." It is certainly sufficient to make very good decisions.

Whether you have chosen to nourish your baby with breast milk or formula, now you have to take care of **sleeping**. The sleep duration and its quality are just as important as the nourishment. If you ask me, between a breastfeeding mother who doesn't prioritize sleep versus a mother who nourishes her baby with formula and at the same time takes extra special care of her baby's sleep – I truly believe (and there is wide research evidence) that the advantages of the formula with sleep are preferable to breastfeeding without care for sleep. In the research list at the end of the book you can read about the importance of sleep and the link between nourishment and sleep in babies and children.

# The Baby Cried and Cried and Cried

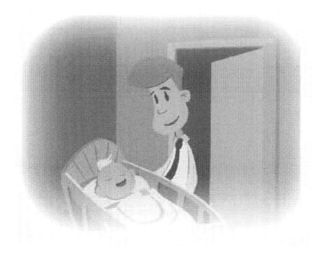

Crying, crying, and crying. The issue that most concerns parents. All we ever want is for our baby not to cry. Crying always bothers us. Crying is interpreted as suffering, and sometimes it is due to suffering.

In this chapter you may find out a few new things about crying, and certainly my personal opinion regarding the crying of babies and children, especially regarding sleep. In fact, if babies didn't cry when being put to sleep, this book would not have been written, and it's possible that sleep coaches and counselors would not be needed either. Parents would put their babies to sleep one way or another and that would be the end of that. The problem starts when you put the baby or child to sleep and **he or she cries**!

When I say "problem," I mean that for the parents this is a problem. I actually see it as an opportunity, not a problem, and let's all face it: Your baby cries every day (and quite a bit). If you are one of those who will tell me, "This isn't true. He actually doesn't cry at all," but he also doesn't sleep, then you surely are just holding him in your arms for hours or performing all sorts of actions in order for him not to cry. If your goal is to avoid having your baby cry, then you are on the right track.

The goal of reading this book is to create healthy sleeping habits for your baby or child, so we cannot be distracted by crying. When your baby cries because he or she prefers to play rather than have his or her diaper changed, or because he or she prefers sweet tea to milk, you do not allow this crying to get in the way of what you think is right. This means that there are things that your baby will want that you realize conflict with what actually needs to be done.

To illustrate, I will use the EIER Model:

The model is based on ideas from psychologist Alfred Adler's approach, and its purpose is to understand human behavior. It helps me a lot in understanding people who operate differently than I do. As a psychotherapist I use this model as a therapeutic tool as well, to better understand my patients' subjective perception and also to teach them how to understand their environment. This environment includes their spouse, their children, their colleagues, and even their friends. In this book I will use this wonderful model to illustrate how different parents interpret events differently, including their child's crying. The acronym EIER stands for Event, Interpretation, Emotion, and Response.

**E is for Event:** The origin of the event is external. The person has no influence or control over it, and that it why it is objective.

**I is for Interpretation:** Understanding the event. This is a cognitive process which occurs in the mind of the person who has been exposed to the event. The process is internal, which is why it is a subjective stage.

**E is for Emotion:** The feeling that develops within the person following the interpretation that he or she attributed to the event. The process is internal, thus subjective.

**R is for Response:** The automatic action which a person is used to performing following the appearance of a particular emotion. The process of the reaction is internal, thus it is also subjective.

The reaction of a person to an event which he or she has experienced will thus be determined by a process comprised of cognitive, emotional and unconscious mechanisms. When the process is understood and clear, a person will be able to separate the process into its components, to examine it, and if need be, to influence it so that the end result will match his or her desires.

**Our Event:** The baby's crying.
In this case the crying is the event. In the vast majority of the cases we have no control over the event. It just occurs. Babies and children sometimes cry. They cry for different reasons and this is their way of expressing a need or a discomfort. By way of example, when the issue is sleep, some of them have a hard time parting with their parents and taking leave of the day's enjoyable activities. It is likely that you enjoyed it mutually. Now, as it is time to go into a dark room and go to sleep alone, as far as the baby is concerned it is an adverse change in his terms and conditions. Babies express this by crying. By the way, babies cry more when they're tired.

**The Interpretation:**

I have found that many parents interpret their child's crying as pain, suffering, anger at the parents, sadness, or discomfort. The parents express their interpretation of the crying using sayings such as: "Maybe something is bothering him? If I leave her alone, might she feel abandoned or develop a feeling of abandonment? Maybe we are not identifying what it is that is hurting him." One mother even told me that she felt that the baby was crying because he doesn't love her. This was an interpretation that was not reasonable to me, but that was her interpretation of the crying. What determines parental behavior is, of course, the interpretation of the event by the parent.

Your baby is crying because he or she **needs to sleep**. It's as simple as that. The child has an unfulfilled need and is crying because he or she is tired! The baby needs to sleep but does not know how to do it. He or she has already played, received love, hugs and kisses, finished eating dinner, and is tired. Very tired. And sleeping on his or her own is a skill which he or she has not yet acquired. There are many adults who also suffer from sleep disorders. They toss and turn and it takes them a long time to fall asleep. The reasons for sleeping difficulties in adults are many and varied (and I won't get into it in this book), but one of the problems may be bad sleeping habits from infancy and childhood.

Your baby is now in a process of growing, developing, and learning many new skills. One of these is the skill of sleeping. Every learning process involves discomfort and frustration. We all know how difficult it is when we learn a new language or new skills at work. It is never easy. It always requires effort and training. It usually requires stepping outside of our comfort zone.

Your baby is in a process of learning to sleep independently and is expressing frustration in his or her own language, which is crying—"I need to sleep and I still don't know how to do it." So instead of stopping for a moment and thinking about how to help with the acquisition of this new skill, some of you just pick them up, rock them, jump around on a physio ball with the baby and perform the falling asleep process with and for him or her. This is short-term thinking, and what we call "putting out fires."

Life is a marathon, not a sprint. In parenting we must consider the long run as well. Tomorrow is another night and the baby will again express difficulty and frustration at the falling asleep process, and again you will need to pick up and rock him or her. So why wait for tomorrow? Come tomorrow, you will (best case scenario) again need to bounce around on a ball. There are babies who succeed in the sleep process only when one of the parents puts him or her in the car and drives on a bumpy road for at least a few miles. I have a surprise for you – as the child grows, he or she will need more and more miles to fall asleep and there will come an age when this will no longer help at all. You will grow weary, and you both will be very tired and impatient. It's a very frustrating stage and it is accompanied by guilt over your expected anger. I suggest avoiding this outcome altogether.

I've been there as a young mother. My daughter would only fall asleep in my arms. She was 2 years old and weighed 33 pounds, and I was desperate – that is where the struggle over sleep started for us.

I was exhausted. She was fortunate that I loved her more than life, but I have to admit that there were nights that even this greatest of love was of no help to me. I was screaming, I don't know at whom or for what. I was desperate. You have no idea how much I would so like to spare you what I went through. The anger was unjustified. She was not at all to blame that I had accustomed her to falling asleep only while being held, but I had reached my limit. I was suffering from lack of sleep, which resulted in a low threshold for frustration, irritability, stress and an inability to function at work.

Let's look at it from the opposite standpoint. Here's how I **don't** interpret the baby's crying when put to sleep:

- He or she isn't suffering
- Nothing is hurting him or her
- He or she is not experiencing fear of abandonment
- He or she is not helpless
- He or she is not all alone in this world

He or she is just tired and crying over it, due to the need for sleep and the frustration over not being able to fall asleep. The child is unable to fall asleep because during the first few months of life (and it does not matter if it's the first 3 or the first 18) you have put him to sleep and he didn't do it on his own. The child is addicted to the nipple, or to rocking, or to being held, or to a bumpy ride in the car. It's not your fault, but it is your responsibility. You did it because you did not know better.

When parents ask me, "Maybe my baby is crying because something is hurting him?" I say, "Maybe."

If your baby is sick or was ill, or was injured, or had an operation, he or she might be in pain and in need of a pain reliever. But when a healthy baby has had a wonderful day, taken a bath, and is now tired – nothing hurts. He or she is crying because **he or she is tired and needs to sleep**.

Let's imagine for a moment that something is actually hurting your baby. Maybe a new tooth is coming in and it is bothering him or her. If that's the case, give the child a pain reliever (one that he or she is not allergic to). A baby doesn't hurt every evening right at bedtime. If he or she was really hurting, he or she would be crying all day, in which case you should see a doctor. But doesn't it seem strange to you that the baby laughs and claps and smiles all day long, and only at night when put to sleep starts crying? Aren't you just smiling to yourselves now and saying that I must be right? Come on, admit it, and let's be done with that.

The baby really isn't a helpless creature. **Not at all**. He or she possesses amazing abilities. And while a human baby doesn't possess the colt's ability to stand on its own feet right after birth, and while he or she is entirely dependent on the parents or other significant adults for care, the baby is not a helpless creature.

I am always amazed at babies' never-ending ability to learn and develop, including the ability to learn how to fall asleep independently. This does not mean letting them learn it on their own, just in the same way that they cannot learn to walk or go up to the fridge and take a bottle on their own.

I wholeheartedly believe in the method that I have developed, which is based on my professional experience as a certified nurse, midwife, and psychotherapist. The method that I have developed for the baby to put itself to sleep and sleep the night through is a routine that a baby will adopt within an average of three nights. When followed correctly, the parents don't get in the way of his process, but rather respond to the child according to the guidelines and with absolute consistency. They help the baby learn how to do it on his or her own.

My method does not instruct that you put the baby in bed, walk out of the house, and let him or her cry. Absolutely not. Any baby's crying, at any age, needs to be responded to, regardless of whether it's from pain, frustration, or even indulgence. The parents must respond and the big questions are: How? When? How much? And this is where there are great differences between the different ages, health conditions, and lifestyles of the parents and the child. The purpose of this book is to be an effective guide to exercising the method which I have developed to teach your baby or child how to sleep.

Now, after we have recognized the Event, a baby's crying, and we've seen how this event can be interpreted differently, we are at the

Emotion which the Interpretation raises.

**The Emotion:**

For some parents the feeling that arises following crying is pity. A mother once admitted to me that many times the feeling that was aroused in her was anger – all day she would give herself to this 12-month-old baby, gave up a career to raise him, and she sometimes felt anger because he wouldn't stop crying.

The emotion which arises in me when the baby cries before being put down to sleep, or during the process, is just a feeling of responsibility. When the baby cries because he or she is tired, I feel that I have a responsibility to teach him or her to sleep so that he or she can easily transition from one sleep cycle to the next without interrupting the sleep process. I am not upset with the baby and I don't feel pity, I am just happy that, after 3 days on average, he or she will put him- or herself to sleep for 10-12 hours nonstop all through the night. The baby will feel that he or she has responsible, stable and strong parents who put him or her down to sleep when the need arises.

Don't get me wrong: It isn't easy for me to hear a baby crying. It instantly affects my emotional side. My stomach cramps with discomfort because it isn't fun to see, and especially to hear, a crying baby. They are so sweet, and it is so much more pleasant to hear them laughing. Crying is a very unpleasant sound to anyone. But I pull myself together and activate my rational side. To act from the rational side doesn't mean acting with no emotion. I realize that the moment in which the baby cries when put down to sleep is a moment during which he or she expresses his frustration, "I need to sleep but I don't know how to do it. For three months or more I was put to sleep by being cradled in a parent's arms, or while nursing, and now I need to learn how to do it on my own." It is very frustrating.

In my opinion, proper parenting combines both the emotional and rational aspects of our minds and hearts. I love giving the example of my parents who were very nurturing during the day and took care of all of our needs, and when it was time for bed it was very clear to us that at night, we sleep. My mother used to say: "I too deserve some rest." She would also make sure she took a daily afternoon nap.

As a mother of five (born within eight years), she put a great deal of time into doing things for us – cleaning, cooking, driving us to after-school activities, telling stories, taking us to playgrounds, etc. – but she knew how to take care of her own needs as well. The most prominent of them: sleep. More specifically, an afternoon nap and a continuous night's sleep. There were five of us, and we all slept.

The message was clear: You will receive everything that you need. At night we sleep! And as I can attest for myself: I never experienced fear of abandonment, I never had pains at night, and I was never a miserable or helpless child. I was a child who learned a lot of things, experienced a lot, acquired many skills, and slept wonderfully (except for the periods when I made the terrible mistake of putting my children to sleep in my arms and in the car).

I have no idea why I did not do what my parents did. When we are young parents, some of us want to be like our parents, and some of us try to do exactly the opposite. In my defense I will say that in those days there weren't any sleep coaches or guide books. We had to engage in trial and error.

You will have a much easier time if you diligently follow the instructions for this fabulous process. Put your baby to sleep in bed and don't take him or her out of it. Why? Because he or she needs to sleep. You will soon learn what should be done in order to help with the learning process, but for now it's important to emphasize what not to do: don't take the baby out of the bed, don't rock the baby in your arms, don't put the baby to sleep with the help of milk, don't bounce on a ball, and don't drive around with the baby in the car. All you do is put him or her in bed (with a hug and a kiss).

I know that's a lot of "don'ts" but it's only temporary. You will soon get detailed instructions as to what to do decisively and diligently.

**The Response:**

Now that we have examined the crying Event, the individual Interpretation, and the Emotion that these interpretations evoke, we reach the fourth stage of the model: Response.

In fact, our response to crying is in accordance with our Interpretation and the Emotion following it. When we feel pity, all we want to do is make that unpleasant feeling go away. When parents act only emotionally, they tend to make mistakes. In parenting it's important to act rationally most of the time. This does not mean that emotions should be excluded or that you shouldn't be sensitive to the child's needs. Not at all.

The response of the parents who interpret their baby's crying as he or she lies in bed on the way to sleep as being miserable will be different than those of parents who interpret that it's simply time for sleep and the baby too should make an effort to put itself to sleep, taking an active part in the learning process. Different reactions will have different results.

In fact, in the last stage the R can also stand for Results. The parents' reaction will have an influence on the pace of the baby's independent sleeping-skills-learning process, and a certain discomfort is part of the process. What is important to stress is that the response should be consistent.

Even if you decide not to respond in accordance with the guidelines of this book, your response still needs to be consistent. Babies and children do not like change and inconsistency. It confuses them. Their confidence is built in part by rituals and repetitive events. This is why it's important to have a more or less regular order to the day, one that was created according to the baby's needs and not that you sat down with a pen and paper and decided on. Babies and children like to know what is expected. When parents are inconsistent, they interrupt the process of calm and peaceful sleep.

The response of parents working according to the "Shhh…at Night We Sleep" method is very consistent. The child or baby is very clear on what he or she needs to do and what the parents' response will be. There are no surprises. The response depends on the baby or child's age, and sometimes other factors as well, like the number of other children sleeping in the room, whether the child is sleeping with its parents, whether you are planning to teach the child these skills at home or during a vacation, at the beginning of the week or on the weekend, etc. All these factors influence the outcome and you will to learn what is expected of you in the upcoming chapters. What is important is that you, the parents, will act in exact accordance with the instructions, with determination and consistency. You are the teachers. It is never what the baby does, but rather only your reaction which is of significance. The baby can do many things— cry, laugh, toss and turn in bed, suck his or her thumb, stand up in bed, call out names. The child is allowed anything. You, the parents, have but one thing to do: respond according to the guidelines of the method.

**Important to know:**
Crying is not an ordinary part of my method just like breast congestion is not an ordinary part of the breastfeeding process.

When one does not handle breastfeeding in the right manner, congestion is created.

So it happens, that when one does not conduct a proper daily schedule for the child, and especially if the child is put to sleep when he is over-tired and not in accordance with his sleep windows, he goes to bed and cries.

Notice that when your baby is hungry, and you delay feeding him (for any reason), he will cry so hard that even when you already give him the food, he will eat it while crying and irritated.

When a baby is hungry and fed on time, he opens his mouth (sometimes even with a smile) and just…eats.

What I am proposing in the "Night is for sleeping" method is that you fulfill your baby's needs…on time.

The result: within a day or two he will gladly go to bed. We all want to rest our head when we are tired, and bed is the best place for it.

Your baby waits to get to bed when he is tired just like he waits for the nipple or bottle when he hungry.

Remember: it's NOT important what the baby does. It IS important how you respond.

And another thing: Your baby is not a guinea pig. The "Shhh…at Night We Sleep" method is not to be tested on the baby or child. You either do it, or you don't. If you just try the method on your child and decide that it isn't working for you, or you don't like it, it will be very hard for you to teach him or her something else. The child will feel that you are not serious and with a little louder crying he or she may lead you to do things you know aren't right. It's not a process which will enhance his or her well-being.

I suggest that you read this book closely. Maybe even read it twice before you begin. But when you make the decision, DON'T TRY, DO!

## Windows of Sleep

When a door closes – a window (of opportunity) opens, and I recommend coming in through it – into bed.

During the day we all take part in different activities. Babies tire very quickly and there is a great deal of energy that goes into every seemingly insignificant activity. Babies from birth until (about) ten months of age, have windows of sleep created every 20 to 45 minutes correspondingly. For those who are already 12 months of age, a window will open after an hour of intense activity. When the window of sleep opens the baby does not seem happy about it. He will look tired, rub his eyes, yawn and be generally unpleasant to his surroundings. That is the exact moment to put him to bed. That is the time that his body needs sleep and is ready for the falling asleep process.

If during this window of opportunity you have not put your baby to bed, he may yawn and rub his eyes a while longer and then he will magically start smiling, laughing at you, and you (naturally) will get enthused, smile back at him and there you have the "perfect" recipe for taking a child out of his sleep time. If you try to put him to bed now, he will put forth a great deal of energy to show you that bed is no longer right for him at this time.

Parents who will insist will make him to go to sleep, but the process may be prolonged and will include a great deal of crying, which will cause him and you significant stress in the process. I am not concerned about a baby's crying when he needs to sleep. But if the crying is because he was put to bed when he was not tired or when he was overly tired – I object to it, because it is unpleasant for both parties. Either way, the need for sleep is critical and very important even if you missed the window of sleep, but in order for the process to be pleasant, short and easy, it is advisable to enter the window of sleep right when it opens. The process of the window of sleep opening may take a few minutes so when you identify it, pick up the baby, give him a kiss and a hug and put him to bed for some sweet sleep.

Do not stress, parents quickly learn what the baby looks like around the time of the window of sleep. Within a few days you will become experts on the subject and be the architects of your baby or child's sleep.

If you missed the window of sleep and you do not want to put him dawn with crying or unpleasantness, just remember the known law: Life is a supermarket... you pay for everything. He will not get the rest he needs, and he will be tired, cranky and irritable, but you will then muster up the almost never-ending parental patience that we have as parents.

# In Practice – What Do We Do?

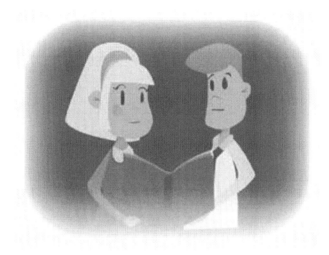

Equipped with all of the information regarding food, bathing, and sleep, we can start teaching the baby and child the practical, independent sleeping-through-the-night skills.

We the parents are here, and you have to sleep. Those are the two messages at the basis of the "At night we sleep" method.

Two short, clear, simple messages.

How can we relay the message to the baby that we are here and yet he or she needs to sleep? That is the art of it and it will be achieved by diligently sticking to the method. Each age group has its own specific characteristics, therefore I will split them into two major groups, with each group divided into two subgroups, based on the child's age.

1.  First group
    1.1  3-5 months
    1.2  6-11 months

2.  Second Group
    2.1  12-24 months
    2.2  2-5 years

At each age and under any condition, we will accompany the baby or child to bed with a hug and a kiss. That's how a good night's sleep starts. If your baby or child immediately puts his or her head down and slips into the falling asleep process that is wonderful. You are one of the lucky ones who does not need a method to teach your child to sleep. If you are parents to a baby or child who is having a hard time shifting from day to night, I invite you to join me on an exciting journey of teaching your child to sleep!

Every night is the end of a day. The child's physical and emotional state during the day impacts the night's sleep process. That's why it's important to provide the baby or child with all its needs, which include food, touch, love, play, and enthusiasm during all the wonderful things that he or she does in the process of growing and developing. A baby who receives all that during the day most certainly can (and should) sleep through the night.

Parents ask me, "When does the night begin?"

There is no clear answer. It depends on your daily schedule. And yet, I really love 6 PM as a time to end the day. In the winter, it's possible to start preparations for sleeping by 5:30 PM because it's already dark outside, and in the summer you will probably prefer 7 PM or 8 PM because 6 PM feels like the middle of the day.

One way or the other, you are the ones who will choose the time you want to start ending the day. When you have decided, try to keep this as a permanent time to begin the process. Usually it's about half an hour before the baby gets into bed.

## The Continuous Night's Sleep: The Six Steps

*Step 1*

**The house turns into a Hall of Sleep:** The atmosphere of the day needs to change. In order for that to happen, the following steps must be taken:

**Decreasing light:** when the amount of light around the baby is decreased, it increases secretion of melatonin (the darkness and sleep hormone) from the pineal gland. There is a low level of melatonin secretion until the age of 2 months, which is why babies can hardly differentiate day and night. But starting at 3 months of age these levels rise gradually, reaching their peak at around 5 years of age, then decreasing slowly throughout the rest of one's life.

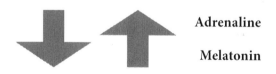 Adrenaline

Melatonin

**Decreasing external stimuli:** When stimuli decreases, the levels of adrenaline (arousal hormone) also decrease. Turn off all electronic devices (TV, radio, cell phone ringtones), pick up the toys, and speak softly to the baby. At first this will seem strange to you, speaking softly to a 3-month-old baby (and even to a 6-month-old baby). But when you turn this tone into a habit in the evening, the baby will grow into a child who will know and be ready for the sleeping process as soon as he or she hears you speak differently than you do during the day.

The tone makes the music.

You would be surprised, but our tone of voice as parents also has an effect on the children's quality of sleep. Starting at the time of dusk, I recommend lowering your tone. Don't shout. Don't put the entire household under stress. It's late and we need to get to sleep. It's better to sleep an hour less than have the children get into bed with the sense that their parents have lost control. A better option is to start preparation for sleep an hour earlier and calmly.

These actions will help your baby or child shift from day to night. This is both a physical and a mental preparation. It's about hormonal changes which occur as the light goes down. As it starts getting darker, the levels of melatonin rise, as the amount of stimuli decreases, the levels of adrenaline drop. Babies and children have a hard time with transitions and the right intervention at this stage can help with the transition to sleep.

## Step 2

**Supper:** We have already learned the principles of supper. Remember that in the room you and the children eat, the atmosphere needs to be pleasant and the room well-lit.

## Step 3

**The bath:** Remember that the bath needs to be short, practical, yet pleasant, and should be given by one parent, not two. I request the presence of one parent, as I noted in the chapter about the bath, so that the baby does not feel like he or she is parting from the whole family. It's easier to go to sleep parting from one parent than from two.

If there are additional children in the house, it's best to bathe the child you are teaching how to sleep before the others or after them. A joint bath might hinder the sleeping process. We can save the advantages of the joint bath for the weekend.

*Step 4*

**Entering the Kingdom of Sleep:** After the bath, you most likely put clothes on the baby in his or her bedroom. There are parents who prefer to diaper and clothe the baby in another room, and that's okay too. Your comfort is very important, but still it is preferable to dress the baby in its own room so that it is clear that this is where he or she stays to sleep.

As for the pajamas, I recommend that they be half a size larger than the baby's size so that it is comfortable to move in. A pajama which is too tight will inhibit the baby's ability to move its arms and legs easily, an important part of his or her ability to warm him- or herself up. The bedroom needs to be dark, with a small night light (which we will turn off eventually). As a rule, the dressing of the baby will also be done by only one parent for the same reason I gave in the previous chapter.

The International Health Organization supports putting babies until the age of 12 months (and especially until the age of 6 months) in the parents' room, but not in the parents' bed. If your baby sleeps with you in the same room, then the entire process should take place in your joint room.

*Step 5*

**The Parting with the Toys Ceremony:** We move on to the parting ceremony from three toys or three pictures in the room: "Good night to teddy bear, good night to dolly, good night to the bunny and… Good night to you (the name of your baby)." When there is a nightly parting with a smile from the set toys, a routine is created that babies love. There are those who are used to singing a lullaby and there are those who pray. To each his own. The principle is to have the activity be short and not one that could raise adrenaline levels.

*Step 6*

**Entering into bed:** You place the baby in bed with a hug and a kiss and you turn off the light (the night light as well). Even a small lamp in the room can inhibit the production of melatonin and cause disturbances in the sleep. Mosquitoes are also attracted to light sources and we would not want them to bite the baby. Make sure that moonlight does not enter the room, and at dawn not even an unwanted ray of light. Only around 6 AM will the window be opened, the light allowed to come in, and with it love, hugs, kisses, and breakfast, stimuli and games and…love, love, love. Lots of love. Because when the baby feels loved and safe during the day he or she will sleep better at night.

If you are one of those lucky parents who puts your baby in bed and he or she immediately puts his or her head down and starts falling asleep independently, you may skip the next few steps. It's wonderful and there are parents who will feel jealous, but if you are like me, who did not have this happen with any of my three children (what a pity there wasn't any baby sleep counseling or coaching in those days), then you should follow the instructions step by step in order to teach your child the sleeping skills.

### Dos and Don'ts

There are things you want to make certain you do:

Allow the baby to independently enter into the sleeping process, which might take about half an hour, during which he or she could mumble, make noises, or move around in bed. During this stage do not enter the room, thus allowing him or her to put him- or herself to sleep.

If the baby cries for a full minute, go into the room (barefoot or wearing shoes which do not make any noise), touch him or her on the arm or on the back and say, "Shhhhh," then immediately leave the room. During this stage the baby might start crying louder, and this happens to many babies who were born to nurturing parents. They feel you, know that you are next to them and so naturally may cry more. The child, though, doesn't want anything **other than to sleep**. He or she does not need to eat at this stage, does not need safety, nor love, or games. **He or she needs to sleep!** He or she does NOT need to be picked up. He or she does NOT need to be rocked. **He or she needs to sleep!** They don't know they're in a learning process, and it will happen quicker than you might think. I assure you it will happen if you are precise, adamant and consistent.

After you have quietly left the room, and only if the crying persists, you go in every minute, touch him or her, and say the mantra "Shhhh," then immediately exit the room. There is no limit to the number of entrances, and the emphasis is on you not staying in the room with the baby. Your presence is only getting in the way of his or her falling asleep. Think of yourself trying to fall asleep with someone walking around the room. You also shouldn't hide right outside the room. During this minute, continue your regular activities in the house. No need to keep the house perfectly quiet – you do not need to worry about flushing the toilet in the restroom, for example. I wouldn't, however, throw a party at this stage of the baby's learning process. There will come a time when a party outside the child's room will not bother him or her. It all depends on your precision at this stage of the process.

When do we stop going into the baby's room? When one of two things happens:

- The baby will suddenly stop crying
- The baby is still crying but it is subsiding

If one of these events occurs, you should no longer go into the baby's room. Just like that. Don't go in. If you go in again and again to the room after the crying has died down or stopped, you may replace one conditioning with another, i.e. you'll replace being put to sleep with rocking by being put to sleep with touching and caressing.

If after a minute or two the baby goes back to crying and complaining, do not go back into the room. Allow him or her to put him- or herself to sleep with the aid of the Transitional Motion, which I will share with you momentarily.

And if the baby keeps crying for an extended period of time? Should I go in?

The answer is: No. After there has been a decrease in the tone or the crying has stopped, you do not go back in.

I understand the difficulty of not going back into the baby's room after the crying comes back. If this instruction is not just difficult for you but actually impossible as far as you are concerned, and will still be that way after you have finished reading this entire book, then don't use this method and look for another option which will suit you better. I don't suggest any other method to parents. I teach the method that I have been investigating, learning, and teaching very successfully for 18 years around the world. Sleeping is a significant and central part of the physical and mental health of children (and of yours, the parents). To sleep is healthy, and sleep deprivation is illness, in the short term and in the long term. The "Shhh…at Night We Sleep" method is one which is compatible with 100% of the babies and children, but most certainly not suitable for all parents. I trust you, parents, to make the right choice for your child and your health according to your beliefs and the information that you have. The ultimate goal of this book is to teach your babies and children the basic skills of **sleep**.

Let's go back to the stage where the baby has gone back to crying. At this stage the baby might cry for a while and there is no going back into the room. During the stage when you were going into the room and touching him or her while saying the mantra: "Shhhh," he or she received two messages:

- Sensory, feeling: **We are here**.
- Behavioral: **It's night time... We sleep**.

You went into the room any number of times as long as the baby was crying constantly and continuously. The moment he or she stopped crying or the crying subsided, you stop returning to the room, even if after a few minutes he or she go back to crying.

The purpose of not going back in after the crying has stopped or subsided is to allow the baby to find its own endogenic (internal) motion with the purpose of self-soothing. Some call it a stereotypic motion, or the self-soothing motion. I call it the "transitional motion". It's the motion the baby does to calm itself down.

Many years ago it was discovered that babies have the ability to soothe themselves and that every baby adopts a specific motion to regulate his or her emotions. We are referring to the selfsoothing motion. The soothing motion usually involves hands, mouth, ears, or hair. At the sensory level the movement involves elements of touch, pressure, or vibration which may manifest in head shaking, eye rubbing, blanket fondling, or a rhythmic touching of one's own body.

There are numerous advantages of using the self-soothing motion, and the most significant one is the baby's ability to regulate its mood even during times of colic and other times he or she is feeling discomfort due to growth and development. In my method, I use the baby's congenital ability to soothe itself and shift from one sleep cycle to the next while utilizing this wonderful motion. During sleep, a baby who has learned the use of the self-soothing motion may go back to sleep independently when shifting sleep cycles. There is research evidence that babies who learned to use the self-soothing motion grow up to be children who are better able to control their own tempers, to be less impulsive, and able to achieve a higher level of concentration at school.

When the baby cries during the falling asleep process he or she is expressing frustration, "I need sleep but still don't how to do it without help. Up until now you have rocked me in your arms, or mom or dad put me to sleep on a car ride because the bumps in the road helped me fall asleep quicker and better. Now my parents read some book and expect me to fall asleep on my own. This is a breach of contract with life! I need sleep, and you need to put me to sleep. This is how it's been for three, or four, even five months and now you expect me to learn something new?" Yes, dear beloved baby, during the first 3 months, while your stomach was still small you needed to eat day and night. What could we do? You got used to falling asleep while nursing and getting milk. Sometimes, if you had a hard time falling asleep, we, your parents, interpreted your crying as you feeling miserable and helped you go back to sleep with a pacifier. We did not consider that you would need the same thing every sleep cycle and that we would be exhausted and start arguing between us about who would get up in the middle of the night to give you a pacifier, or milk, or to rock you. But today, when you are over 3 months old, weigh over 11 pounds and have improved your abilities, especially the ability to sustain food in your stomach for 10-12 hours, your needs during the night have changed. It is now only a need for sleep. We expect you to sleep a full night and trust you to succeed. And don't worry, you aren't growing just thanks to nourishment at night. At night you continue growing with the help of the secretion of the growth hormone from your pituitary gland. In order to learn this skill (today we all know that it is a skill which needs to be learned) **we are here to help you**.

**So how can you help your baby?**
When you diligently and precisely carry out the instructions of the "Shhh…at Night We Sleep" method, your baby will learn how to put him- or herself to sleep and sleep a 10-12 hour night straight through.

Please don't say, "I wish." It's not "I wish." It will happen! There's only one condition for success: that you do everything that I ask of you without any deviation at any stage, and then you will discover that your baby is able and capable of falling asleep independently and sleeping through the night. What is most important is not to try this method on the baby. Just do it. Do or don't. There is no trying the system. I remind you: Your baby is not a guinea pig. If you can count on your determination, consistency, and precision, **Start! Today! This evening! Tonight!**

There are parents who will need help or coaching. Sure, with this book you can do it by yourselves step by step, but if you decide that you want to read the book and then do it with coaching, contact a sleep coach who is knowledgeable in the "Shhh… at Night We Sleep" method. You can ask for recommendations, search social networks, Google, or go to my website at www.sleepallnightusa.com.

If you are reading this book in the morning, start teaching your baby how to sleep this morning. If you are reading it at noon, start with the afternoon nap. If in the evening, then start in the evening. Just don't delay the learning process. Every day of continuous sleep is important for your child as well as the rest of the family. The beautiful thing about this method, in addition to all the advantages I have already listed, is that you can start the process anytime, even at 1 AM, when you are tired and feel that all hope is lost.

A 3-month-old baby is expected to sleep about 10 hours; and from the age of 6 months they need and can sleep 10-12 hours consecutively. In fact, I teach babies to put themselves to sleep starting on the first day of their lives. In the beginning of life, the stomach is small and unable to hold food for more than 2-4 hours, so babies need to be fed during the night as well.

During the night it's a mistake for parents to turn on the light, change a diaper, hug and kiss (hard not to, I admit!), feed, walk around for a while – sometimes hours – so that the baby burps, thus wasting hours the baby should be sleeping, it gets used to the evening activities, and that's where sleeping disorders can start for babies and children.

This book deals with the issue of babies' sleep starting at the age of 3 months, but it is certainly possible to teach babies good sleeping habits starting on the day they are born (while nursing the baby during the night according to its needs).

**Consistency is an inseparable part of order, which is so important for babies and children. It helps you, the parents, to set boundaries, and it helps babies and children know what to expect and what can happen at any given moment.**

Now, some things to avoid:

Don't TRY the method. Either DO it or don't do it.

Don't get into situations where the baby falls asleep in the stroller or while feeding, especially during the week of the learning process.

Don't start the process before reading the entire book and studying the instructions carefully.

Don't expect caregivers to perform this process at daycare, unless they have read the book and are well-versed in all aspects of the method. Daycare teachers have their rules and regulations and trust them not to inhibit the process even if they do things differently at daycare. Don't worry! Babies and children very quickly recognize that things are done one way in a certain place and differently in another place. The important thing is that both places have consistency.

Don't perform the method in part, just in the same way that there is no "half pregnancy."

While the "Shhh…at Night We Sleep" approach is a method for teaching babies and children how to sleep a full night, we all know that sleep during the day affects sleep during the night and vice versa. Sleep brings sleep. So how do we help our babies and children navigate the naps they require during the day?

## Day Sleep

The baby can be awake between an hour to an hour and a half, and then needs to sleep again. At this time, he or she will start showing signs of tiredness, and a window of sleep opens which should not be missed. Starting at the age of 3 months babies slowly start differentiating between day sleep and night sleep. They are aware of the wonderful things which occur during the day. They are adored, smiled at, and played with. They will not easily take a break and go into a dark room to sleep. You can help the baby go into the day sleep by gradually lowering the level of activity, dimming lights by closing the shutters, and putting your cell phone on silent. Create a pleasant sleep time with less stimuli so that the baby doesn't feel that he or she is missing out on something that is happening right outside their room.

It is important to put the baby down when he or she is tired, but not too tired. When the baby is put to sleep in an overtired state, he or she has trouble falling asleep despite the fact that he or she really needs it.

Most babies will sleep three times during the day: Morning (about an hour-and-a-half), noon (about an hour-and-a-half) and afternoon (between an hour to an hour-and-a-half). It is important to point out that during the day sleep cycles are shorter and many babies wake up after 20-40 minutes. Theoretically, they are supposed to go back to sleep for another sleep cycle, but in fact, some parents interpret the waking between cycles as waking up and take the baby out of bed, despite the fact that the baby is still tired and needs another cycle of sleep. This baby will be yawning, red-eyed and restless. The reason is that he or she woke up for just a moment between two cycles and needs to go back to sleep, but the parents interpreted the waking as the end of the nap. The correct thing to do per the method is not to take the baby out of bed, and to react the same way we do to shifting between sleep cycles during the night: wait a minute, and if the baby doesn't go back to sleep independently, go in, touch him or her, say, "Hushhhh," leave the room, and allow him or her to go back to sleep to complete the new sleep cycle. Some babies will take time to go back to sleep between two cycles.

It is my experience that the process of teaching the baby to learn how to transition between cycles during the day may take up to a week. There are parents who will prefer to take the baby out of bed due to its difficulty to shift from one cycle to the next during the day. To those parents I say that this is an okay decision to make. The baby may stay tired, not smile as much but will get used to shorter sleep cycles. It is not preferable, but possible. I leave this to the preference of the parents. Obviously, I would choose to perform the process during the day and the night the same way because sleep during the day affects the sleep at night. Babies that sleep well during the day make it to the night more relaxed and calmer, and thus sleep much better. Tiredness during the day negatively affects the night sleep, so it's best to keep the sleep routine going during the day as well, and preferably in a quiet and dark place like a bedroom.

If you have caught the moment when the baby is tired but not too tired (what is sometimes referred to as the "window of sleep"), there is a high probability that he or she will go to bed without crying at all. If the window of sleep has passed and he or she is overly tired, there is a chance that going to sleep will be accompanied by crying (normal crying, which will pass when you allow him or her to fall asleep independently). This is the price that you both pay for the fact that he or she went to bed overly tired. That's okay. It's not fear of abandonment and it will not affect the baby's emotional state, not in the present or in the future. When the baby is hungry and not given food on time, he or she also cries for the nipple. This is the price for being late in feeding the baby, and this, too, is not that terrible. You just need to always make an effort to supply the baby with his or her needs when he or she needs them. I know many adults who, when they are hungry, it is best to stay away from. The same goes for babies and children. When they are hungry or tired, rocking will not help, and if it does, it will be only for a short period of time.

It is important to allow babies to be alone a little bit, too. They look wondrously at everything around them. Everything is new to them and they learn to enjoy what they see around them. Even if it isn't a special activity, they get tired after an hour to an hour and a half.

When the baby gets into bed overly tired and cries, and you allow him or her to fall asleep on his or her own, you are doing the right thing. You are allowing the child to learn the skill of falling asleep independently. Don't beat yourselves up and say that it isn't his or her fault that you got him to such a state of tiredness. It's okay if falling asleep takes a little longer than usual. When the baby wakes up, he or she will find a smiling mother who will come to him or her, pick him or her up in her arms, and ask with a smile, "Who slept so beautifully?" And he or she (at this age a social creature by now) will smile at you and you will melt. That's a promise.

Don't look for a daily schedule at this age. This is the age when you have to follow the baby's needs and identify when he or she is hungry and then feed him or her, and when he or she is tired, you put him or her to sleep, and when he or she needs a hug and play time with his or her parents, and also when he or she needs to be by him- or herself. Starting at this age babies should be taught how to occupy themselves. A baby who can occupy itself will reach the age of five without constantly complaining "I'm bored." Teaching the child to occupy itself is to be done from birth. And if you don't agree with me that this skill needs to be taught from day one, let's compromise on 3-5 months. Beyond this age, habits are formed and there is no force stronger than habit. It's harder to teach a 5-year-old to teach him or her to play by him-or herself.

*How will you identify your baby's window of sleep during the day?*

- Timing: You need to catch the moment at which your baby starts showing signs of tiredness (a yawn, eye-rubbing, whining)
- A decrease in body movement and energy
- Motions that he or she makes to soothe him- or herself, such as putting a thumb in his or her mouth or touching a soft toy to his or her face.

*How will you identify that your baby is not sleeping enough and has sleep disturbances?*

- Yawns a lot during the day
- Looks tired, especially around the eyes.
- Falls asleep in all sorts of places like on the play rug, during a drive in the car, and during a walk in the stroller
- Falls asleep on a regular basis on the breast or while nursing from a bottle
- Crying a lot during the day

## Characteristics of babies ages 3-5 months

Starting at 3 months of age, babies already have a routine that parents have created for them. As for sleep, there is a chance that an undesirable routine has been formed. Even where little babies are concerned, most of them have been able to acquire bad sleeping habits. In this short period of time, breastfeeding is already well established and easier on the breastfeeding mothers and the nursing babies. For the bottle-nursing babies, the required amount of milk stabilizes around 3.5-7 oz. in every meal. Parents who choose to start giving solid foods at 4 months will have a nice addition beside the bottle.

Remember that babies need to acquire trust in the world. They need touch, love, kisses, and also to be adored. Communication should be encouraged, and they need to be exposed to stimuli such as toys, voices, and even mutual playing. The determination and consistency need to revolve around the sleeping. Between sleep times, pick them up, hold them in your arms, and kiss them a lot. It's important to remember the combination of touch and love, all the while remaining strict regarding the baby's sleep. This is the ultimate combination for raising a physically and emotionally healthy baby.

At these ages you can no longer excuse the crying as gas, either. The babies' digestive system has grown and gotten used to life outside the womb, and generally babies in this age group are calmer. It is already expected that they put themselves to sleep. If the baby cries when he or she is put in bed, and the rest of the time smiles when he or she plays, you can be certain that your baby is addicted to your arms, the breast or the bottle as a means of falling asleep. It isn't possible that he or she smiles on the play rug without any gas and then when he or she is put in bed all of a sudden gas appears, right?

At this age, babies already voluntarily smile at familiar or smiling faces. This makes babies prefer the presence of their parents for sleeping to being alone in a dark room. These are normal reactions for a healthy baby. At this age the baby experiences difficulty falling asleep in a changing environment, especially in a place with a lot of stimuli.

## Characteristics of babies 6-11 months

At the age of 6-11 months, the baby is already eating solid foods in addition to breastfeeding or formula. Solid food stays in the stomach longer, so the babies can and should sleep around 12 hours consecutively. These are conclusions derived from research studying the emptying of the stomach for the purpose of giving medications to babies and children, which is why it is best that supper includes solids and not just milk. During the day babies can be awake close to two hours before they need to sleep again.

Starting at the age of 6 months, babies will already enjoy playing with their parents much more, but there is no need to be attached to them all the time. Full supervision yes, but occupying them only partially. It is very important to give the baby time to be with him- or herself as well. Babies at this age are in awe of everything around them. Some of them already crawl and use up lots of energy, and within about two hours will start showing signs of tiredness: yawning, eye-rubbing, or starting to nag.

In the evening you will find that babies already protest having to part with you. Despite being tired, they might show difficulty in separation, especially babies closer to the age of 12 months. The baby already understands the advantages of staying and playing with you, and will not be happy about ending the wonderful day with you. It's important to remember that sometimes the difficulty in parting is mutual. These are sweet babies whose company you've enjoyed during the day. This is an age at which babies spread smiles and rolling laughter all around and it isn't easy to end it all just like that, but we have no choice. The baby needs his or her sleep so that tomorrow he or she has the same wonderful disposition.

In order to end the day, stimuli and games must be decreased gradually and shifted into a calmer atmosphere which includes dimming of lights, speaking softer, stopping the playing and singing, and telling the baby what is about to happen. Yes, even a 6-month-old baby understands the tone and meaning of your speech, much more than you can imagine. One day your baby will simply respond.

Around the age of 8 months your baby might be able to stand in the crib on his or her own. If this happens when you are in the process of teaching the skills of falling asleep, remember that you should not go in and put him or her down if he or she is standing in bed, but rather follow the instructions. Attempting to sit or lay him or her down might require force (and that we do not want to do). Furthermore, we don't want to start a conditioning process in which "if I stand up in bed a parent will come in to put me down". Just go in, touch, and Hushhh!

## Babies aged 12-24 months *(who sleep in a crib because it provides him or her with boundaries and safety)*

If your baby is in the 12-24-month age range and is still in a crib, I'm glad.

As for the timing of moving the baby to a transitional bed, I recommend it when one of these occurs:

The baby is unsafe in the crib because he or she might jump out (you observe him or her attempting to get out on his or her own).

The baby is weaned off diapers and thus should be provided with a safe and easy way to get out of bed when he or she needs to go to the potty.

It has been my experience that babies have a harder time learning how to fall asleep in a transitional bed before the age of 20 months. If your baby has not reached that age, it is advisable to heighten the rails of the crib for safety.

Babies at 12-24 months already know how to do many things.

Parents are already set as "objects." This means that even when the parent is not next to them, babies are aware of the parents' existence. When you play "peekaboo" with these children and hide your face behind your hands, they will wait for that "peekaboo" and know that you are there behind those hands. They love this game because, at this age, children love to predict what is going to happen. There is a very structured routine here, one that they have created from infancy. They and their parents already know each other well.

Usually these babies have already learned to walk. There are 12-month-old babies who have already been walking for a month or two, and there are those who will walk independently only at 18 months.

If you have accustomed them to playing a little on their own, they will be able to occupy themselves for as much as half an hour. And if not, they will want you to participate in the toy festival around them. I love babies at all ages, but there's no doubt that 12-24 months is my favorite. They are already "little big people" and more interesting to be around.

Day sleep is important at this age as well. Around the age of 12 months there is a need for two naps during the day, and at around two years of age they will usually need only one. In each case, it isn't advisable to give up on day sleep. If the midday nap is prolonged into the late afternoon hours for some reason, you should not wake the baby up so that he or she sleeps better at night. It's a big mistake to wake up the baby. We never know what part of a sleep cycle he or she is in, and he or she might wake up cranky and upset, and rightfully so. If sleeping in the afternoon is not a habit, this will not get in the way of sleeping through the night. And even when this occurs, the household should still enter a sleep mode around 6 PM.

If I still haven't managed to convince you, or you have a different experience than what is described here, and you do decide to wake up the child after he or she has slept enough in your opinion, then please make sure that you wake him up not by talking or touching but rather with opening a window, turning on a light, and waiting for about 15 minutes. He or she will most likely wake up at the right time in the sleep cycle. If you make sure of that, he or she might even wake up with a smile, stretch their arms and legs, and be ready for your hugs and kisses.

For the learning process, carefully follow these instructions:

First go back and review this chapter if needed.

The first five steps apply to this age range too.

The first steps we've learned:

1. Turning the household into a "hall of sleep"
2. Dinner
3. Bath
4. Parting with the Toys Ceremony
5. Putting the baby into bed

Children at this age enjoy many things along the day. They've discovered new things, learned about the world and had fun. Don't expect them to say "Dear parents! Thanks for a lovely day.

I understand everything eventually comes to an end so let's say good-bye to this day with hugs and kisses and have a wonderful rest of the evening." That won't happen. I promise that!

You should, however, turn the house to a "hall of sleep" around 6PM and decreasing stimuli (picking up toys, turning off the TV, talking softly), the baby will understand the next stage it getting into bed and... sleeping. Within three days in average – you might not believe it but it will happen, he'll prepare his body to bed already when saying good night to the toys.

Until the baby gets used to falling asleep alone he or she might show resistance of being put in bed and left alone, and will show that with complaints and protests.

If he or she cries for a full minute, go into the room, quietly (barefoot or with quiet shoes), touch arm or back, say: "Hushhhhh… It's night… now we sleep!" and leave the room. If the baby stands in bed do not sit him down. You repeat the same mantra whether baby lies down, sits or is standing.

At this stage the crying might increase, and that's natural. The baby would probably like to continue with the happy day or being put to sleep with a previous method that put it to sleep. But today **you want something different, something better**. You want to allow the baby to fall asleep alone so it could move between sleep cycles without an external aid, which will allow a nonstop good sleep with all its advantages.

Fortunately, the "At Night We Sleep" method only takes three days in average. Remember that your baby is put into bed after a day full of love and activities, as well as dinner. At night a baby doesn't need to eat, feel safe, love or play. Only to sleep! He or she needs you to allow them to sleep. Not to be rocked, only sleep! A baby doesn't know it's in the midst of a learning process and that will happen faster than you can imagine. You only have to be precise, determined and consistent.

After quietly leaving the room and coming back every minute, but only if the baby keeps crying, touch him or her and repeat the mantra: "Hushhhh…" and immediately leave the room. You do that until the crying stops or subsides. Either of them mean the baby has found his or her soothing motion and that will help them fall asleep on their own. If you keep coming into the room you might disturb its using the motion and implementing it. If the baby starts complaining again you do not reenter the room and let the baby find the soothing motion, the transitional motion. The motion done by the baby soothes him or her, instead of relying on an object like a pacifier or cradling by a parent.

It's their own motion and it's always with them. They will never lose it and will always use it if you let it.

During the day your baby received all its needs, physically: food, cleanness (bath); and mentally: hugs, kisses, playtime and learning. Before putting the baby to bed you have a parting ceremony from the toys. Now it's time to sleep.

When crying – you go in, touched the baby and repeated the mantra. As long as it's needed. Not more than that. More than that will only hurt.

He'll search (and find) the transitional motion and fall asleep by himself. A connection in the brain will be made between the motion and falling asleep on its own, The next day the connection will be automatic. Yes, just after a single day. Or maybe a couple of days. Only when parents are imprecise does the process take about a week. Of course, if you're fumbling the whole thing your baby will never learn to fall asleep on its own. I trust you to be precise because that's why you're reading this book.

Remember that your presence in the baby's room only harms the sleeping process. Think of yourself trying to fall asleep with someone walking around the room. Don't hide right outside the room. Babies have special sensors. They're very sensitive and know a lot more than we give them credit for.

You, the parents, are expected to go on with your regular activities around the house. The baby's learning process depends on your accuracy.

As I mentioned in the previous chapter about the baby standing up in bed is the same for this age group. If a baby stands in bed you should follow the same instructions without laying him down. The baby will soon lie down and enter the sleeping process on its own. You will be very happy.

**Children ages 2-5** *(who are sleeping in a transitional bed or in a youth bed)*

As background it is important that you read the chapter "In Practice – What Should We Do?" The first three steps are applicable to this age group as well.

- Turning the household into a "hall of sleep"
- Dinner
- Bath

Children 2-5-years-old are no longer babies. They are children. They know many things, have learned many skills, including many social skills. They know how to stand their own ground, their verbal abilities improve daily, and it is advisable to include them in everything that you see fit. They have the ability to play with themselves and with others. So you should listen to them, they have lots of interesting things to tell you.

I'd like to say a few words about the special age of 2, which is similar in its characteristics to adolescence. It's no wonder it's called in the literature the "adolescence of childhood". At this age children discover they have new abilities and they can make certain things happen. They start expressing their will and won't take "no" for an answer. The best way to act with this age group is to avoid power struggles. It's important to hug them while setting borders. Sleep is non-negotiable. Sleep is needed just like food, like going to the bathroom, and this is what needs to be explained to them, plain and simple.

Children between the ages of 2-3 still need one nap a day, usually around noon. I recommend not waking up a child from at this age range either, even if the nap is prolonged. If you have decided to wake him or her up from the nap anyway, please make sure that you do so by opening a window and turning on a light, not by touching and talking, and then wait 15 minutes for his or her spontaneous waking. Chances are he or she will wake up at the right time in the sleep cycle. If you are diligent with this, the child might wake up with a smile, stretch his or her arms and legs, and be ready for your hug and kiss. Starting at 3 years, though, most children will not express a desire to have a nap. They just have a lot of things they need to take care of, they are very busy.

Some parents tell me their child doesn't like to sleep. "When I ask him if he wants to sleep, he always says no." I would like to inform these parents that children don't always know how to say or show that they are tired. Their ability to judge situations such as hunger and tiredness can be lacking. It's a parents' role to identify these situations and get them food or to bed. They can seem cranky. When you ask them if they are hungry, they might say that they aren't, but in fact after they eat they will be calmer. The same goes for tiredness. 2-5--year-olds are already "big" kids, but when it comes to sleep (and food), the parents are still the ones who need to take responsibility, to identify tiredness and hunger, and make sure their needs are fulfilled.

**How can we help them learn to fall asleep and to sleep through the whole night?**

Even when talking about ages 2-5, it's important to put the household in sleep mode an hour (at least) prior to bedtime. The children are full of energy, playing and running around and the levels of adrenaline (the arousal hormone) are very high at the end of the day. I suggest talking to them in a lower tone of voice, decreasing the lighting in the house, and preparing them for the fact that soon they'll have dinner, followed by a shower and bedtime. Children like to be prepared for what is about to happen. We don't like having plans sprung on us either. As part of the respect that children deserve, we must inform them about what is about to happen.

I suggest you refrain from starting new activities with them close to bedtime, simply start shifting down gears instead. Reading a book at this hour is a great activity that might be pleasant for both you and them. In the beginning they might not understand the meaning of the "quiet talk" in the house and might put you to a shouting test. Some children will cooperate and speak softly, too, and some may purposefully talk loudly or even shout. Remember, don't preach to them to talk quietly. They still haven't read this book. It doesn't matter what they do but the way you react. If they shout, you respond quietly. For example, if your 3-year-old is yelling, "Where is my ball?" you will quietly answer, "I think it's under the bed." You don't bring stress into the house, especially not at night before bedtime.

After dinner and a bath, they need to brush their teeth and have a short parting ceremony with you and/or other members of the family (this could also involve parting from the toys or a lullaby). Some children are used to having a story read to them as part of the ceremony and that's okay. There are children who will ask for a story and a song and a parting ceremony from every object in the house. Most children at this age will do anything, and I mean anything, to delay going to sleep. They just want to prolong the day. At this stage there is a conflict of interests between the parents (who want to end the day) and the children (who want it to go on). The fact that the parents want to end the day is not just because they have had enough and they're tired (although there are those who will admit that it's a little of that too), but most parents understand the importance of sleep as a component of their children's physical and emotional well-being.

When the child is in bed, you say good night with a hug and a kiss. There is a chance that if you prepared your child to the idea that each person sleeps in his or her own bed after a hug and a kiss, he or she will simply fall asleep within minutes. If there is no problem, there is no need for a solution. In case you expect the child will soon call for you again and start demanding your presence, you need to act as follows:

Let the child go on to his or her own into the sleep process, which might take about half an hour, during which he or she might move or talk in bed. Do not go into the room during this stage and allow him or her to put themselves to sleep.

If he or she calls you, go into the room quietly, say: "Hushhh… it's night time… we sleep!" And leave the room.

If he or she gets out of bed while you're still in the room, walk towards the door and only when you are out of the room, hold the child's hand and take him or her back to bed as you say the mantra: "It's night time… we sleep!" In your regular voice, never in anger.

If the child keeps getting out of bed, keep putting him or her back repeating the mantra, "It's night time… we sleep!" It's very important to take the child back to bed only by holding his or her hand. Do not pick him or her up and do not kiss and hug him or her. Because as long as the child benefits from getting out of bed, he will keep getting out and will not go to sleep. In the child's mind, he or she needs to get out of bed in order to receive your love. It's wonderful to give children love, warmth, and touch, of course, the more the better, but only during the day! At night, we only sleep. Night is not the time for attention and love. Your child has received everything he needs from you during the day. We mustn't forget that children are born "businessmen."

Wherever there is a gain to be had (e.g. attention), they will utilize all the tools at their disposal to achieve that gain.

This is how you should escort your child to bed as many times as required: Go into the room, put him or her into bed, say the mantra, and leave the room. This process can be exhausting, for you as well as the child. When you perform it precisely every day for a week to ten days there is a great chance that the child will no longer want to get out of bed, because what's the point? If there is no gain, there is no point in making an effort. It isn't worth it just to hear you say the mantra. But

146 | FROM SUNSET TO SUNRISE

if after a day or two he or she says, "I want to eat," and you respond, "You have already eaten dinner," or "Tomorrow we'll eat breakfast," or any other answer deviating from the mantra "it's night, we sleep," he or she might realize that there is room for negotiation.

There is no need to give the child food if just a short while ago he or she finished dinner. Even if you think that he or she didn't eat enough, they'll make up the calories in the morning. This way the child will learn that it's best to sit at the table and eat, because when you leave the table at the end of the meal "the kitchen is closed". It's okay to not allow the child to do to you what is called in the professional jargon "access operating". If you start going back into the kitchen or answering questions on different matters, he or she will not easily give up on a dialogue with you during these beautiful hours of the evening. You can go about your household business, no need to keep everything perfectly quiet. You do need to remember that if there is extra noise or excitement, the child may feel he or she is missing out on the grownups' action. I recommend that while putting a child down to bed, continue with your regular activities but lower your tone and try to keep things relatively quiet.

At the beginning of the process the child might not understand what is going on. Until now you have sat next to him or her in bed, read one to dozens of stories, and all of a sudden you expect him or her to get into bed, not come out of it, and fall asleep on his or her own.

You can explain to children from the age of 2 and up what is about to happen, and it's best to explain what is about to happen from now on, as opposed to what happened before today. The explanation should be done in the early afternoon hours and not just before they get into bed to sleep. Sit with them away from screens and cell phones and give this conversation your undivided attention. Every parent knows their child, and will explain this new idea of independent sleep in accordance with the child's age and maturity. The idea for all ages and for all children is to explain that you read a book that a "sleep teacher" wrote, and she explained why it's important to sleep well. "Mommy and Daddy need to sleep well at night, too, and we need your help. The sleep teacher said that the room needs to be dark (because it's better for a good sleep and also when there is light the mosquitoes come to bite). Everyone needs to sleep in his or her own bed until morning and Mommy and Daddy go to their own bed, too."

Don't expect the child to happily accept the fact that from this day on he or she needs to get into bed and fall asleep alone. The child's job is to test boundaries and resist, unless you present the issue as one that was meant to increase the child's worth due to the fact that he is already a big kid and you trust him or her to succeed. If this works and the child accepts the idea with understanding, remind him or her again at dinner. If he resists, be empathetic and explain that there are times when we need to do things that don't seem as fun but need to be done. Sleep is required. For you as well as for us.

A couple told me that their 3-year-old son was constantly preoccupied with who was the strongest kid in kindergarten. After he expressed anger and objected to the idea of sleeping alone in his room, they sat at the computer with him and searched the internet for "sleep and muscles," and showed him pictures of people with muscles sleeping. The child went to bed and said, "Goodnight, I'll wake up in the morning with strong muscles."

Be creative and find the right words to explain to your child why it is important to sleep. You can also explain why you need sleep. Parents need to drive a car to all sorts of places, to prepare food, to work. They need energy, which is received from food as well as from sleep. Take the time to explain and guide your child, and perhaps you might earn their cooperation and avoid unwanted power struggles.

At this age, as in any other age, it is important to give the child attention and quality time during the day. A child who has not gotten his or her needs fulfilled during the day will make any effort to win your attention at night. When there's more than one child in the house the atmosphere and dynamics between the house members is important. Try to create a pleasant atmosphere based on mutual help, cooperation, and a feeling of belonging for each of the family members. When the children feel valued and feel they have a good place in the family, they will go to sleep more relaxed.

At older ages, sleep disorders are a function of bad habits acquired from infancy or created when a new child is brought into the family. In cases like this, the older child loses his or her place and then discovers that the attention which he or she was used to getting during the day, he or she can get during the evening or night when the baby is asleep. When you identify the link between the birth of a new baby and the beginning of sleep disturbances of an older child, two things should be done:

Provide the older child with attention and a sense of belonging during the day. This, of course, does not mean over-attention, but rather concentrating on him or her while he or she is doing positive things, and coming up with things to do together.

When the older child tries to get attention during evening and night hours, don't fall for it. Be pleasant and practical. Say goodnight. If you are used to reading a book or singing a lullaby together, make sure you keep this wonderful ritual and no more. End it with saying that tomorrow you will meet for another day together. If you start doing things that you have not done before because of his or her demands or your guilt over bringing a new sibling into the family, you might hinder the sleep process and his or her peace of mind. You don't have to be tough, simply be consistent.

# Fear Will Keep Mommy and Me Together

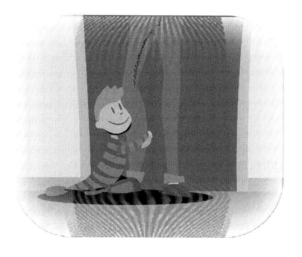

By the time they turn 3, children already possess a very rich world. They know very well how their parents will react to what they say or do. They know if you are negotiable on almost everything, including the going to sleep process. The Adlerian approach says that children have good goals and wrong ways of achieving them. Among their good goals is the need to feel a part of a family (and later wider circles), and the need to feel as though they are contributing and beneficial.

If the child is pleasant and cooperating during the day, and the parents are attentive and encouraging, there's a bigger chance the child adopts the behavior during the day and won't need to do it during the night.

Fears are always born in children accidentally. When a child first says that he or she is afraid of monsters, thieves, witches, or anything else, the parent immediately stresses. Wow, the child has fears! The parent's reaction to the first time the child expresses the word "fear" will largely determine the fear system that the child will suffer from for days, weeks and months to come.

The word "fear" frightens many parents. What does a parent do when he or she hears their 3-year-old indicate that he or she is afraid? Try to answer the question yourselves.

I once asked my parental coaching students this question and these were their varied responds:

- Try to find out what the child is afraid of
- Ask the child if something has hurt him or her
- Tell the child that there is nothing to be afraid of and sit next to him or her until he or she falls asleep
- Allow the child to come and sleep in the parents' bed until the fears go away
- Leave the child a night light and calm him or her by explaining that if the monster comes the child should come to the parents' bed

The answers given by the students were not particularly good. They are possible, but each has a price which I am not sure you would want to pay.

It isn't reasonable that fears come to a child who has played and functioned normally during the entire day just at the moment the day ends and it's time to go to sleep. This doesn't mean that the child is not experiencing fear. Of course, he or she is, and it is real. But **the real fear is a purposeful fear**. The goal is for mommy to remain next to me. The child learns very quickly that if he or she says to his parents "I'm afraid," they will immediately focus on him or her, and the child and its fear become the center of attention. Fear is the means by which the child obtains attention just as it is about to end with the day.

**So, how do you treat this fear and allow the child to sleep with a full sense of security?**

This is where the parents need to give up on their personal fear and stand strong before the child. First when the child expresses the fear they need to show empathy: "I understand that you are afraid. There are things which really scare us. But when we have a fear, we need to overcome it. Tomorrow in the morning we will each talk about our fears, because mommy and daddy are afraid sometimes too."

A mother who came to me for parental coaching told me that after she was coached on how to handle her 4-year-old daughter's fears, she told her daughter about how she herself had overcame her childhood fear of snakes. Then her daughter said to her, "I am afraid of burglars, and you know how I overcome it? I check that the alarm light is on every day." The mother wonderfully encouraged her by saying, "Wow, good for you. It really helps that there is someone who makes sure that we don't forget to set the alarm," and a conversation about the alarm system began, and then home insurance, and so on. From that night on, the child parted from her mother with a kiss and the fear was no longer a means of getting the mother to stay with her until she fell asleep.

As a rule, I suggest not to worry when the child says he or she is afraid. If it's a fear that appears only at night, this is a hint that the child has found the means to keep you close and receive more attention. If the child is also afraid during the day you need to find out what the source of the fear is. Sometimes a child has had a traumatic event and then you need to seek professional assistance. When "regular" fears show up, you should talk to the child, share some of your fears and talk about the fact that fear is natural and normal and just needs to be overcome. Fear is a normal emotion and evolutionarily it protects us from many dangers. For a long time after my youngest got her driver's license, every time she left the house and got into the car I would say to her, "Be afraid! When you are on the road, be afraid of drunken drivers, of traffic violators." I scared her about what could happen if a driver answers his or her cell while driving. It's okay to be afraid under certain circumstances. Of course, when fear paralyzes us or the children, that's a different story, and then we should figure out if there are any underlying goals intended to keep the parents at the child's side and perform the falling asleep process for him or her (also referred to as secondary benefit).

Then there is the occurrence of nightmares, which are dreams from which the child wakes up alarmed. The child can usually tell you about the dream, and sometimes may not be able to differentiate between the dream and something he or she thinks really happened. In these cases you need to talk to the child, caress him or her, explain that it was just a bad dream and that he or she can go back to sleep. It is a normal occurrence that actually happens starting at the age of 3 and continues throughout life. We sometimes wake up from a dream. Children don't have a clear distinction between their inner world and reality, so the prevalence of nightmares increases (especially at the ages of 3-5).

You shouldn't hinder their sleep routine or develop special ceremonies centered around the nightmares. Don't question the child on what he or she dreamed about, and he or she should be put back to sleep as quickly as possible. You shouldn't talk about "what happened last night" the next day either. If the nightmares recur nightly, try to find out if something's going on at daycare or find out if there was an unusual event that left an emotional impression on the child, and then treat it directly.

**Did you know?**

*Some children sleepwalk or sleep-talk. When sleeping the speech is unclear and usually incoherent. The child, of course, is not aware of the talking and doesn't remember it. Sleep-walking is unconscious and can start with talking in bed and then going out on a nightly "stroll" through the house. In cases like this, you should make sure there aren't any objects on the floor in the child's way so he or she does not trip and fall. As isolated events, sleep-talking and sleepwalking are rare and are no cause for concern. It usually stops by adolescence. This is a normal occurrence unless it repeats itself often, and then it's advisable to seek advice and treatment. These occurrences worsen during times of stress and sleep deprivation. Sleepwalking is also attributed to children who do not have clear boundaries.*

# Even When Sick – At Night We Sleep

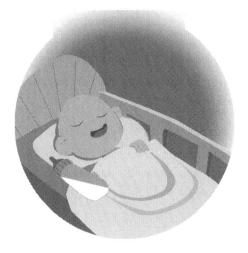

A sick baby is a very unpleasant situation and justifiably knocks the parents off balance. The routine is interrupted, the baby's behavior unexpected. He or she is fussy and generally looks miserable.

When my children were sick, I was under a great deal of stress. It seemed like the end of the world to me. I felt a need to only pamper them to make up for the fact that they're sick and not feeling well. That's why I perfectly understand parents who lose it when their child is sick.

I am so excited to share with you what I wish I had known back then to spare you the suffering I experienced.

Now I know that when a child has an illness it isn't a tragedy. Healthy babies and children do get sick. There isn't a child who hasn't gone through an ear infection or an eye infection, or diseases such as the measles, mumps, chicken pox, etc. Except for extreme and rare cases, these babies and children are sick for a few days and then they recover. With a little bit of rest, natural or conventional remedies, and airing out of the room, the child gets better.

It's important to know that during illness, **sleep is twice as important**. During sleep, the body receives the rest it needs and the immune system works more efficiently. When we are sick and lose our appetite, the energy which was meant for the digestive system is directed at healing the body.

Food should not be given at night during illness, either. Water, yes (very little) unless the body temperature exceeds 100.4 degrees (F) and there's diarrhea and vomiting, which mean loss of fluids. Then fluids, water or tea, are essential so that the baby does not dehydrate. No milk or food of any kind. Yes, even if the baby has not eaten during the day, **nighttime is not for eating**. I am, of course, talking about the ages of 3 months and up, despite the fact that at these ages it isn't advisable to give water. Water can fill the stomach and decrease the number of calories that the baby will take in during the day. But during an illness I suggest only giving your child water at nighttime. If there is a different medical indication, I recommend you follow it.

When a pediatric surgeon came to consult me about her 9-monthold baby girl's sleep, she had a hard time accepting the recommendation not to breastfeed at night. She sadly said, "How will she survive the entire night without nursing?" She realized that after a night or two the baby will get used to it, but expressed a concern regarding the first night. I asked her what she asks of parents of a baby this age, or even younger, a day before an operation. She said with a smile: "8-12 hours of fasting, depending on the type of surgery." I asked her, "And the babies survive that night?" She smiled and said, "Obviously." Nothing bad happens to the baby or child even if during an illness they don't

156 | From Sunset to Sunrise

eat during the night. Only good things happen, including nonstop sleep during which the brain (the part called the hippocampus) and the immune system operate without disruption. Rocking in your arms is not a solution or a remedy for ear or throat infections. On the contrary, when the child is sick he or she needs to be in bed and sleep. When you pick him or her up, you are getting in the way of sleep and delaying the healing process.

Another thing that I learned and is an important message to all parents: A child is not miserable until pitied. If we take care of the baby or child according to what they need and not consider them as miserable, and not treat them as if they were miserable, then they will never be miserable. I love to give the example of one of my good friends whose child was born with a genetic condition and, starting at the age of 6 months, required regular blood transfusions. She never told him he was miserable. She would emphasize how lucky he was that he had the strength to deal with the transfusions, a loving family, a wonderful personality and many friends that want to be close to him, and that he was an excellent student.

Thanks to that, this child was one of the least miserable children in the world. He sang in the school choir, excelled at robotics, finished school at the top of his class and became an amazing person. It was this friend who taught me one of the most important lessons in life. It doesn't mean not being empathetic, not helping, not listening or not being there to support those in need, but there's a big difference between that and pity. Why is it important? Let us return to the EIER model.

**Event:** The child has a throat infection

**Interpretation:** The child is miserable

**Emotion:** Sorrow

**Reaction:** Constant holding in arms, kissing, giving up sleep habits and more…

Notice that when our interpretation leads to the feeling of pity we prevent or inhibit the recovery of our baby or child. How do I know? Because when the baby is sick he or she needs medicine, fluids, and sleep!

How can we help our child recover faster with the help of the "Shhh…at Night We Sleep" method?

We will also demonstrate with the use of the EIER model.

**Event:** The child has a throat infection

**Interpretation:** My healthy child has a throat infection and needs treatment

**Emotion:** Responsibility

**Reaction:** A visit to the pediatrician, giving pain relievers, insisting on drinking and not food, and diligently sticking to the sleeping routine.

Parents should act according to the situation and problem.

When the sick baby or child has slept enough and wakes up, you can and should give him or her a kiss (if the baby is not contagious), read a story on the couch, go out for a little bit of sun (not too harsh) weather permitting, and air out the house. The fact that the parental response should be rational doesn't mean that we will not take care of our baby or child in a sensitive and loving way, as these two approaches are not contradictory.

---

*Did you know?*

*Continuous sleep deprivation weakens the immune system and your health.*

---

**What do you do when the child is sick?**

When babies and children are sick, you need to decide if you will see a doctor. If you see a doctor and he recommends medical treatment then you should follow it, of course.

If your baby or child is not feeling well, has a fever below 100.4 °F but is nagging and does not have an appetite and you have decided that you do not need to go to a doctor, it would be good to give a pain reliever that you know the child isn't allergic to. Giving medication like this on occasion can do miracles. If his or her appetite is lost, don't insist on food. Do insist on drinking water or tea. Babies over 12 months can have a little bit of honey added if they aren't sensitive to it. If your baby or child has a high fever it's important to check on him or her several times during the night. Set an alarm clock, even though there's a good chance the baby will wake you up anyway, but you can't count on that. High-grade fever needs to be monitored.

During days like this you should keep a natural environment as much as possible and there's nothing better than having mom or dad stay at home with the child until he or she is better. If that isn't possible, then it's better to have a nanny or a grandparent come to the house. Your baby will sleep better in his or her bed in a familiar room. There are limitations sometimes and if the only possibility is to take the child to somewhere else, that's okay. If the caretakers keep a clean environment, provide the proper medical treatment, and stick to sleep times, the child will get better anyway. We can't always do what is best, so we need to function under less desirable circumstances as well.

The important principle to remember as we end this chapter is to stick to the rules of the method even in sickness. No breaking the rules! **Even when sick, at night we sleep**!

Naomi's parents came to my clinic when Naomi was 6 months old. They told me that Naomi was born with a congenital heart defect and immediately after birth had to undergo surgery. The surgery was successful and the doctor explained that Naomi did not require any special treatment. The concerned parents felt bad for their baby because of what she had to go through and after surgery, they simply did not put her down. In their words: "During the day we managed, more or less, because the grandparents helped, but the nights became an endless nightmare. We have not known one single night of sleep. We operate in shifts, each of us holding her on their turn. When we try to put her to bed, she sleeps for a few minutes and wakes up crying, which breaks our hearts."

Indeed, it is not easy when a baby is born with a medical condition, and the tendency to protect and provide 24/7 attention is completely natural. It is important to remember that anything done excessively may cause other problems. Holding the baby after surgery is essential and important. Sometimes it is important to prevent crying following certain procedures. However, when the doctor indicated that from now on the baby should be treated "normally," it was important to start teaching Naomi to sleep in her bed and not in her parents' arms. The parents were concerned that the learning process would involve crying and thought that the baby should not cry. It was obvious to me that this was an unrealistic expectation, because all babies cry, even when they are tired.

I suggested that they consult the pediatrician again regarding the idea of teaching her to sleep, and I was happy to hear that the doctor allowed them to start the process. He also said that he does not know of babies who do not cry, and that when she learns how to sleep, she will cry less. Naomi learned how to sleep in her bed, which we positioned in her parents' bedroom but at a certain distance from their bed. She slept a full 12 hours during the third night of the process. There was no doubt that that was what Naomi needed. She needed a bed, her own space, and parents who let her sleep. Her parents understood that Naomi needed to be in their arms occasionally and receive love and security, but first she needed to eat and sleep.

# The "Tux" of the Method

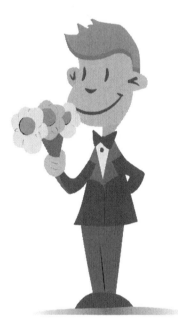

A tuxedo is worn on special occasions, very special occasions.

While there is no need to wear a tuxedo when you are putting your baby to sleep with my system, if parents have a "special occasion" coming up (such as a special Saturday night dinner party) then consistency is even more important in the days that precede the special event.

If you follow my sleep method consistently and precisely each day of the week, there is no reason not to break the sleep method routine for a special occasion. As long as the baby or child is forming good habits through the "Shhh…at Night We Sleep" method, the occasional special event will not disrupt the learning process.

I have a friend who is that way about her nutrition. During week-days, she is very diligent about following her diet, and on weekends she allows herself to deviate because the knowledge of how and what to eat is already embedded in her. She knows how to return to the correct eating guidelines on the first day of the week and each day after.

This is also the right way to conduct things with the "Shhh…at Night We Sleep" method. The method is precise from Monday to Friday, and on the weekend you can all party with the rest of the family members. However, it is important to go back to the regular habits as soon as you return home. In contrast to the diet, we do not wait for the week to begin. Even when the family returns home during the weekend, you need to return to the system.

**Continuous sleep is not to be postponed to Monday**. You can also leave the baby at home with a babysitter, without breaking their routine. It's always best for the baby to go to bed at the time he or she is used to and sleep in his or her own bed. The child will not really be able to enjoy the family outing and be "passed around." Grand-parents probably won't be happy with this recommendation, as visits with their grandchildren are a great source of pleasure. They wait for these wonderful times of family gatherings including all of the older and younger grandchildren, and I can certainly understand them, although I am not a grandmother yet…. This book deals with how to teach babies

and children to sleep and the importance of a sleep routine and learning falling asleep on their own and through the whole night.

It is important that you know that when there is routine – it can be broken. When sleep routine is kept Monday through Friday, it's certainly possible to break it on the weekends. Just remember that everything has a price, there are no "discounts".

This refers to any event that breaks the routine, in which you take the baby with you at a time that he or she is used to be in bed sleeping.

Do what you feel is right. Break the routine and return to is as soon as possible.

---

**Did you know?**

*Parents lose about 350 hours of sleep during the first year of their baby's life.*

---

A mother told me that during the week she stays at home and keeps the sleep routine during the day and night. But every Tuesday she meets a group of girlfriends in a coffee shop, since before they all became mothers. She wondered whether to keep going out to these meetings because she knows that her 6-month-old daughter is paying the price, and yet these meetings were so good for and important to her. She described how her daughter could not fall asleep in the stroller and that many times she needs to hold her in her arms. She asked for my professional advice.

I did not want to make the decision for her but I did tell her what I would do. My answer was: "I would continue to meet with my girlfriends every Tuesday. Not everything that suits me, suits you, too. What might help you with the decision is the cost and benefit associated with every decision. At each such juncture, consider whether the benefits exceed the cost or if you are willing to "pay the price." The price that her daughter pays (forgoing her morning nap once a week) is not that high, and at the same time the mother is happy she meets her friends and does not feel like her entire world revolves around taking care of her baby. As far as I am concerned, the value of friends is very high. We need friends. In many cases they are the source of light and strength for dealing with unwanted situations.

> **Did You Know?**
>
> *Life is like a supermarket – everything has a price!*

The "Shhh…at Night We Sleep" method requires consistency and precision, but a certain flexibility is essential under certain conditions and circumstances – you as the parent will know how to flex and bounce back for the benefit of your baby's quality continuous sleeping process. Our brain can't distinguish between good and bad habits, so if we have a bad habit it will always lurk quietly in the corner waiting for the right time and reward.

Breaking the routine is an opening to a change in the baby's behavior. If breaking the routine has caused you to rock him or her in your arms or in the stroller – the price will manifest itself in the difficulty he or she finds in getting back to falling asleep on his or her own. What is significant about getting back to the routine is the parents' conduct and not the baby's behavior.

What the baby does is not important but how his parents react that counts. When breaking the routine babies might react with restlessness, and the parents need to bring the baby or child back into the routine decisively and consistently.

# Teething and Sleep

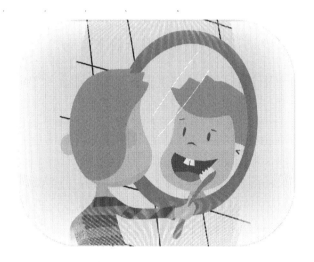

Teething pain is the most common phrase that comes
out of parents to 4- to 12-months-old babies. The baby has diarrhea "because he's teething," the baby isn't sleeping "because she is
teething," the baby isn't eating "because he is teething," the baby has
a runny nose "because she is teething." He has a fever because "he is
teething," an ear infection "because she is teething," is restless because
"he is teething". Teething is blamed for everything.

> **Did you know?**
>
> *There is no research to support the claim that teething causes
> sleep disruptions.*

The baby is miserable because he or she is teething and so he or she is picked up in the middle of the night, fed during times he or she does not need to be eating and put to sleep in someone's arms or in the stroller.

All because of teething!

So, let's set a few things straight about teething and sleep.

First of all, the coming out of the first tooth (it will typically be the lower front tooth) is always an exciting event. I immediately ran over to the baby journal and recorded the event.

**Did you know?**

*Teeth usually come out between the ages of 5-12 months, and the process usually ends towards ages 2-3, then the child has 20 baby teeth, but the process starts much earlier: teeth start developing at the early embryonic stages and are already present in the embryo's jaws (and can be seen in an ultrasound).*

Teeth breaking out and growing do not interrupt babies' sleep. Period. Case in point, there are (many) parents who suddenly find a white spot in their baby's mouth and discover that their baby's first tooth has broken out. There are no "exposed" nerves and no objective reason for pain. Some babies experience a bit of swelling and discomfort, but not pain. The breaking out of a tooth can cause minor rise in body temperature and maybe some restlessness, but there is no link between that and sleep.

If you, the parents, think that the breaking of teeth hurts or bothers, causes fever and discomfort, give your baby a pain reliever. Medications for lowering fever are also effective in relieving pain. Notice the indications on the package: "Relieves pain and… reduces fever",

Let me tell you: these are medications that do not lower body temperature if it's at normal level. Teething pain is a good enough reason to help the baby with some pain reliever. If you are the kind of parent who does not favor medication, find an alternative medicine solution.

Picking the baby up when he or she needs sleep will not make the pain you think that he or she has go away. Giving the baby milk in the middle of the night will not make teething pain go away. Bringing the baby to your bed so that none of you can get sleep is also not a solution that I recommend. I met many parents who acquired many pain-relieving ointments, and I am here to tell you that it is important to check their ingredients. There are ointments that contain ingredients that the Department of Health does not recommend using with children under the age of 2, and even then, it is advisable to consult a pediatrician. There are ointments suitable for use of babies, but should not be given in cases of viral illness accompanied by fever.

> **Did you know?**
>
> *Teething sometimes involves excessive salivation. Chewing hard objects may ease the baby's discomfort.*

**So what do you do?**

If you think the reason for the discomfort is teething, give the baby a pain reliever. If he or she has a fever or any other symptom – take him or her to see a pediatrician so that you do not miss anything that might require medical attention. I object to massaging and touching the swollen area and I trust the baby to know how to put his or her own (sweet) little fists and touch his gums where he or she needs to. It is advisable to take care of hand hygiene. Children discover their hands and other body parts and learn to do by themselves what is pleasant for them. The old adage "Less is more" is appropriate here.

## As for the Night

Put the baby to sleep at the same time, in his or her bed, and if he or she is having difficulty falling asleep, react according to the method. If he or she has (or had) teeth pain, he or she shouldn't suffer twice: both discomfort, as well as interrupted sleep. If you are absolutely determined that this is discomfort which interrupts sleeping, you already know: You can always use a pain reliever. As for sleeping: the same rules apply, the instructions do not change…"because of teething."

A moment before putting your baby to sleep, remember: the baby's teeth need to be brushed from the appearance of the first tooth. This is when oral hygiene starts.

# SIDS

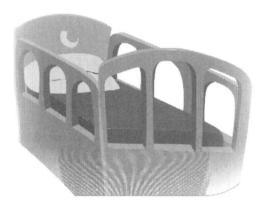

Sudden Infant Death Syndrome is the horror of parents until the age of 12 months. It is a very terrible phenomenon, which to this day isn't understood, despite extensive research that's being done.

SIDS is the event in which a baby is discovered not breathing in its bed. In most cases the baby appears healthy. To this day there has not been an explanation found for this occurrence even with thorough post-mortem investigations.

There are assumed risk factors that have been found to be statistically linked to SIDS:

- Premature birth (SIDS is five times more likely to occur in premature babies than in babies who came to term, 37 weeks and up)
- During winter (probably due to overheating of rooms) and, in

the same vein, rooms which were heated to a temperature of over 77°F
- Babies to smoking mothers
- Prior occurrence of SIDS in the family
- Male babies
- Lower socioeconomic families
- The position of the baby (see below)

There is an assumption that babies prone to SIDS have faulty functioning of the brain and bodily systems that control breathing, temperature regulation, heart rate and the awaking systems, so these babies need a higher level of stimuli to wake up from their sleep to restore breathing. Following research that has pointed to a connection between SIDS and sleeping on the back, a formal recommendation was issued to put babies to sleep on their back and not on their abdomen.

Many parents explain that their baby sleeps better on the abdomen, but still these recommendations should be followed. The rationale behind this recommendation is that babies with higher risk factors do sleep "too well" and their awakening mechanism fails due to their breathing stopping. For babies with Apnea doctors may recommend putting to them to sleep on their back and using a home breathing monitor. The device alerts when a baby stops breathing; the alarm aimed at waking his or her breathing mechanism and also waking up the parents to assist. It isn't always possible to help and there are cases in which, despite everything that was done, the tragic incident could not be avoided.

Such an event can cause a lot of baseless guilt, as well as anxious behavior of the parents with future babies and lack of sleep for fear it will happen again.

It is important to remember that an incident like this is inexplicable, and to this day the precise reason for it has not been found.

Different recommendations are published often and some of them contradict others, so let's hope that research in the upcoming years will increase our knowledge on how to decrease the occurrence of this horrible phenomenon. Still, you cannot fear your baby's sleep. Sleep deprivation or disturbances weaken the baby and may cause a series of health problems. Sleep is a must!

Many parents complain that their baby does not sleep well on its back. These parents are right. Babies do sleep better on their abdomen. Yet until the baby can turn over on his or her own we must adhere to the recommendations of the department of health and put babies to sleep on their back, especially at nighttime when you do not have the ability to look over them.

To prevent the baby's natural reflexes from awaking him or her, I recommend wrapping him or her tightly in a thin blanket, leaving room for a finger (yours), or to block his or her body from both sides with a rolled up towel.

There are parents who put their baby to sleep on his or her abdomen and then turn him or her onto his or her back once the child has fallen asleep. If your baby is already turning over, the instruction to put him or her down on his or her back is no longer relevant. The baby knows how to pick up its head and turn over from back to his abdomen and will do so regardless of how you put him or her down. Most babies learn to turn over from their back to the abdomen at the age of 4-6 months.

In any case, there are measures which are advisable to take to assist in avoiding the phenomenon:

- Breastfeeding has been found (statistically) as one of the factors reducing SIDS. The breastfeeding schedule changes each period. Until recently the recommendation was for up to 6 months and it was then changed to up to 12 months.

- When the baby is awake during the day put him or her on his abdomen for "tummy time" so that he or she has a chance to strengthen his or her shoulders. During the night place the baby on its back. The reason for the instruction to put the child on its back is unclear but the assumption is that while lying on the abdomen, the baby's exhalation is saturated with carbon dioxide and can be dangerous to breathe back in.

- Don't put the baby to sleep in your bed – sleeping with the baby may have disastrous results, such as crushing him or her.

- Choose a sufficiently firm and aired mattress. Firm is better than soft, as is one which is aired to prevent the "greenhouse effect."

- Do not place unnecessary objects in the bed such as plush toys, pillows or other toys. The bed should be aired with no objects present that may block the airway and accumulate dust and dirt.

- Avoid overheating the house, especially the baby's room. It is important to dress the baby in no more than two layers. During summer, one layer is enough, unless there is air-conditioning in the room. The desired temperature in the baby's room is 70-74°F (during the winter up to 77°F, no more).

- Avoid smoking – Beyond the many negative effects which secondhand smoking can cause the baby, it also increases the risk for SIDS. This is an opportunity for parents to stop smoking, but if there is no desire or will to quit, at least don't smoke around the baby.

- Avoid putting in a head protector, and if you do put one in make sure it is not too high. I like a well-aired bed with no obstructions.

It is important to remember: SIDS is a rare condition in which a baby is found not breathing with no plausible explanation.

However, follow the safety instructions in this chapter.

# The Father's Role

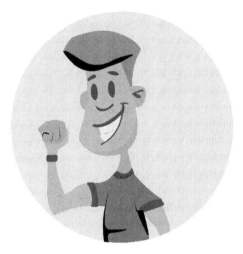

Most of those who seek sleep training for their babies are mothers. Maybe it is related to the fact that they are the primary feeders. Maybe it is because there still isn't (truly) equal division of responsibility between men and women, and the mothers are those who are with the children during the day. Perhaps there are other factors; what is important is the fact that more women seek solutions for their child's sleeping problems than men do. It's a statistical fact. Yet, there is an increase in the number of fathers who take upon themselves the issue of sleeping and they tend to say:

"My wife has a harder time coping with the crying or the frustration of the baby."

In cases like this I always say it's wonderful there is a spouse next to that mother, who takes upon himself the task that is difficult for her. I love parental cooperation. If the mother is having a hard time coping with teaching the baby how to sleep independently, perhaps the father plays a bigger role in sleep training. That is wonderful. It most certainly isn't just a maternal task. Furthermore, I am a big supporter of parental cooperation in child rearing, and the baby's sleeping learning process will be better with both parents supporting the process and walking the path together. A baby or child whose parents are consistent and cooperative in his or her rearing will better and more quickly acquire sleeping skills. If one of the parents objects to a certain method, it is advisable to find the golden path to a method that will be acceptable to both parents.

A couple who came to my clinic told me that they turned to a sleep trainer which the father was apprehensive about, and then turned to me following a recommendation he received at work. The mother felt more comfortable with the first method, but not as much with mine. They decided to follow the first method consistently for one week, and if that did not work, to follow the second one.

I supported them in their decision because within a week a baby should already learn the skill of independently falling asleep. If one method does not work for an entire week, there should definitely be room to change the method. Even though sleep is very important, I do not recommend getting into too much of a dispute over one method or another. I have also found that fathers tend to operate from a more rational place and are less emotional, which is very helpful to the mother, who is often

just coming off of a pregnancy and labor (which were not easy on her) and dealing with issues such as habit-changing and the teaching of new skills to the baby, among other things. It is the husband's role to support, strengthen and be an inseparable part of the process.

Sometimes a mother will schedule a sleep training session for her baby, and when we explain that it is best to come with one's spouse, she says: "I am the only one who puts the baby to sleep… he doesn't need to come."

My recommendation is that the couple comes to the session together. First, it might be an interesting meeting and of value beyond the counseling and the sleep training. The knowledge, research, and the way in which the method was born are fascinating. Second, when the woman will apply what she has learned, her spouse will be able to assist her, practically as well as emotionally. Encouragement always lifts the spirit and promotes success.

Remember: The bond between father and child is essential. Despite the wonderful trend of joint parenting and growing involvement of fathers in the rearing of their children, many fathers still feel useless or unneeded. Experience shows that paternal involvement often helps prevent and resolve children's sleeping disturbances.

**"Two are better than one"**

*- Ecclesiastes, 4:9*

# Single Motherhood

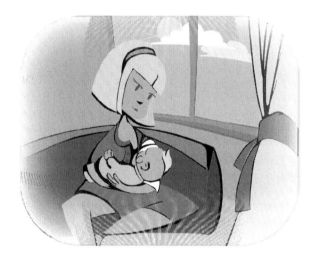

Single mothers make a courageous choice to bring a child into the world without a partner. One thing is sure: these are women who made a difficult choice and who believe that they can raise a wonderful child without a spouse or regular help.

Single mothers face many challenges and yet they are filled with satisfaction when they succeed, raising one or more children on their own. I have met many married women who claim they feel like single moms, despite the fact that they have a spouse. One way or the other, single parenthood is a (poor) excuse for babies' or children's sleeping problems.

I have heard these lines many times:

"I am alone and I don't have the strength to handle her," or "I myself feel that the joint sleeping is good for both of us," or "I don't have the patience to deal with him during the day and the night, so the easiest thing to do is give him a pacifier or a bottle or put him in bed with me."

I understand them all. The solutions these women choose are in fact "easier" but not really so. If that same single mom were to invest three to six days teaching her baby to fall asleep on its own and to sleep a full night, all of the described issues would be prevented and they would both sleep a full night. If you are a single mom – you more than anyone need to solve your baby's sleeping disturbances so that you can gather your strength during the night in order to handle the next day. In many ways, you need to function both as a mom and as a dad. Nothing in our lives is easy.

There are issues of making a living, maintaining health, running a household, taking care of the baby and yourself, and then there are always the unexpected things that just seem to happen. That's why it's so **important that you sleep a full night**. When you have a baby who does not know how to sleep and you do not have a spouse whom you can elbow to get up to go calm the baby – you will always be exhausted. So it is you, more than others, who needs to get it together, follow the instructions, and just teach your baby to sleep a full night.

Single moms also need to learn to seek assistance from anyone that they can count on, even with this process of teaching to sleep. Mom, Dad, grandma, grandpa, friend, sister… Anyone who offers help – accept it graciously. My experience shows that people love to help.

Remember that even if you do not always succeed in seeing it – people will try to do good. If you decided to go to a sleep trainer who works with the "Shhh…at Night We Sleep" method, ask to bring along someone who can help you in the process.

# My Daddy is the Tallest and My Mommy is the Prettiest

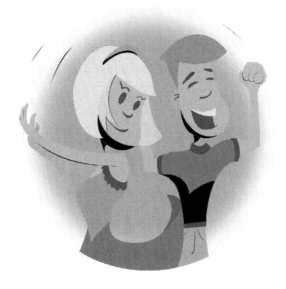

Many parents are willing to sacrifice a lot for the children. Me, too.

The thing is that in order to please the children we often find ourselves doing things that harm us and our health. This is especially common with the issue of sleep. Mothers often tell me that they have no problem waking up a few times a night. They think that's what they should do, and it's true. The thing is: it's true up until the age of 3 months. A sick baby needs special care, including during the night, but babies (thank god) aren't sick 365 days a year, and in rare difficult cases I hope the parents have help. No one can survive days and nights without sleep.

I am referring to those parents who wake up in the night for months, and even years, and not because their baby suffers from a health issue. They don't sleep because their child has not learned to fall asleep on his or her own and sleep a full night, and these parents keep waking up to their children's' frequent waking. This is where the parents hurt their own sleep and thus their health, their appearance, and their patience towards the baby and other children in the house.

Parents who sleep as much as they need to are healthy parents.

Good parents: at night, we sleep!

# The Firstborn's Sleep

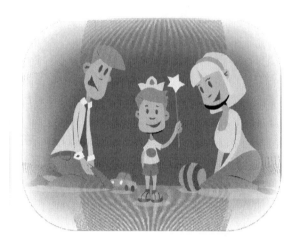

The eldest child has a special status in the family. He or she was born to different parents than those the other children in the family were born to. Immediately at birth, the firstborn became the center of his parents' life. In most families, the birth of the first child pushes aside the couples' relationship in favor of parental roles.

He or she was born to a set of expectations that most likely will not repeat with the other children. A firstborn is expected to bring happiness and achieve greatness. It's no surprise that there are set expectations of him or her that are different than those of the other children. The firstborn can grow up to be the most responsible, the most excelling, the most invested in, and can also be the most spoiled of all the ones to follow.

The firstborn's personality and style will be affected by his or her place in the family (as the first child) and the parental model the child unconsciously chooses (similar to mom or dad).Parents to a firstborn are full of motivation to give and bestow upon their baby everything in their power.

I have heard parents say: "I want to give him everything that I didn't get" and "I want to give her exactly what I had as a child."

In my experience with parents and children I found that parents who were spoiled as children tend to spoil their children (especially their firstborn). Just as they couldn't handle not getting something they wanted as children, they identify with the baby and give him or her everything. And when I say everything, it means that they are constantly busy with addressing what the baby wants and deprive him or her of even a second of frustration.

And why is it so important that children experience frustration every once in a while? Because life is sometimes frustrating, and if the baby doesn't experience this feeling, he or she will grow up to be a child who cannot handle frustration, and then will become a young person who cannot experience frustration. Life is very hard for these kinds of people.

I don't mean for you to create frustrating situations on purpose. I mean that if the (firstborn) baby does not want to sleep because he or she wants to only be with his or her parents who played with him and served him or her all day, the child needs to learn that every day ends. The following day all of this goodness and joy will resume. Parents who want to spare their babies or chil-

dren the little crying or frustrating moments could find themselves frustrated for days, weeks, or years to come. I put an emphasis on the firstborn because the subsequent children arrive into a world in which there is already something very special, so to start with, they are not the center of everything (in most cases). There is already a set of parents and a child, and they are joining a family group. In most cases the firstborn will continue to demand his or her first and special place.

As for sleep, it is very important to know when to draw the line and act as if there is another child in the family. I know this may sound strange and unreasonable. I don't mean for you to walk around the house as if you have another child. I mean for you to just be aware of the fact that in a year, or two, or three, in most cases, another child will be added to the family, and then the firstborn might see him- or herself as a victim because a new baby arrived and will usually replace him or her in the parents' bedroom.

If you are reading this and saying to yourselves, "No way. They will both stay in our bedroom," I don't want to imagine the quadruple sleeping problem that you will have on your hands.

There are cases in which the firstborn is so intent on fulfilling the parents' expectations, that he or she becomes a complacent child. You need to be careful here, too. If you see that your child always wants to do only what you want of him or her, including getting into bed and obeying you, you need to be aware that this child may grow up to be an adult that does things he or she really doesn't want to do, just in order to satisfy the wishes of others. If your child runs to bed and does not object at any stage, be aware and check during the day if at other times and in other areas he or she does everything to be overly compliant with you. In that case it would be a good idea to seek professional guidance. In the sleep domain, it is advisable to encourage him or her to get into bed and sleep continuously because sleep is a health issue and it's for his or her own good, not because you want him or her to do as he or she is told.

There are parents who put their firstborn in bed with them. There is something fun about that for all parties. Think of about it. A sweet child in the middle between two parents. His or her smell, laughter, and joy reaching the sky. Three content beings in one bed. To the parents this seems fun and not too disturbing most of the time. It's even an effective contraceptive. What the parents don't know is that in fact they are at the beginning of writing up the unwritten psychological contract with their firstborn child. The child understands that life is sleeping with mom and dad, and being in the center. "These two people have the role of providing me with attention and love at all hours. If this could go on forever, then fabulous."

The problem is that slowly the baby grows up and the joint sleeping arrangement is less convenient. The parents become less patient due to sleep disturbances, or another baby is born into the family, and then the parents decide that two in bed is too much. They remove the eldest child, who rightfully protests the move, and then the parents think that it's necessary to consult a psychologist. And all this for what? It's simple: there has been a breach of contract with the firstborn. The firstborn refuses to be left out in the cold. He or she needs the warmth and love all the time. Give it, but everything in moderation. And remember that the firstborn is a part of the family group. He or she won't be the center forever, at home or outside. Today you must think about the future.

# Siblings in the Same Boat

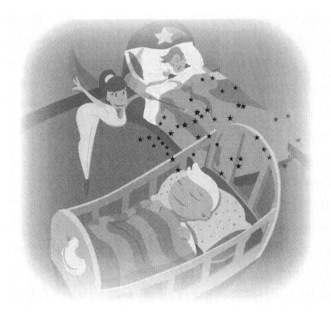

Do not let the title of this chapter alarm you. Sleep is not an enemy. At least, it does not need to be.

Many parents are afraid to start sleep training the baby or child when there are other children in the house. They focus on the fear that one of the children will wake up the other and the child who is already sleeping well could start waking up because of the process that the younger sibling is going through. It's true that the more children there are in the house, the greater the challenge of teaching the sleeping skill. But there is nothing you can do. Sleep is a need and children have to sleep. How shall we teach the baby to sleep when there are siblings in the house? Do we put them to sleep in the same room? Is an additional room required for the baby to sleep in alone? This chapter will deal with these issues.

First of all, if the house is a large enough, it is preferable that each child have his or her own room. I did not have that privilege and my first two children slept in the same room. It's harder to fall asleep in a room with more than one person, and there are more sleep disturbances. If you are lucky and you have a room for each child, start with the baby or child who is going through the sleep training. Once this child is in bed (even if he or she hasn't fallen asleep yet) continue with putting the other children to bed. If you are comfortable putting your children to bed in another order, do that. You know what's best for you.

When two or more children are already in bed, they each should be treated according to the instructions that you have learned. Yes! I can imagine the face that you are making now. "He will cry, she will get out of bed. How the heck do we do it?" The answer is: patiently!

I remind you: You chose to bring children into this world and now there's a period in which they have to learn new skills, such as bringing the day to an end, getting into bed, and sleeping. That is a skill. They are not machines with an on-off switch.

If you get to bedtime relaxed and calmer and with an unlimited supply of patience, the process will be shorter and more pleasant for everyone involved. When I say these sentences to parents in my meetings, they make a face and explain that there is a problem:

"It's the end of the day. We no longer have patience. We gave these children everything and we are already exhausted, wanting to end the day."

I can certainly identify with and understand these parents, and I usually suggest to them to bring the day to a close earlier, while they still have a shred of patience left. Talk to your children quietly, don't be upset with them because you are tired – it's not their fault and not their responsibility. A parent who starts yelling or punishing because the children want to prolong the day is in fact a parent who has broken down in front of the children, which is a hard thing for the child and accomplishes nothing. Get organized earlier. That is golden advice.

And another thing: if you are worn out by bedtime, maybe you did a few wrong things during the day? Children do not need to be hard work, you should work well with them. Did you conduct yourself in a friendly manner with your children, did you include them in tasks that they can help with? Maybe you gave them too much attention so they didn't stop asking for more and more. A parent should not be exhausted. Remember that.

I remember a wonderful meeting with Rebecca, a mother of 15 children (and one grandson).

13 of them lived with her at home.

When I dared ask her how she got along and wasn't she exhausted, she laughed and said: "Dorit, I have 11 more pairs of helping hands at home," (the youngest two being babies who could not help yet).

She told me she already knows at every age what the child can do and from that moment, that's his or her job. She told me she was the queen of the house, and I realized that I may know the theory, but she practices it. That is the entire difference between knowing and doing. When I asked her for an example, she told me that 3-year-old David is responsible for placing the potatoes and the onions in their basket after grocery shopping. 6-year-old Lee takes care of the groceries that go in the fridge. Each child has a role. I learned a lot from this meeting with Rebecca and it changed my view on the role of the parents and the role of the children in the family.

It's no secret that the more children take part in the household tasks, the more they ease the load on the parents, as well as raise significantly their personal sense of value and worth. I contribute, therefore I am! The process of bringing the day to a close and putting everyone to bed is the responsibility of the parents, but the sleep itself needs to be the responsibility of the children. If you give them the responsibility, they will take it. If you don't give them the responsibility for their sleep, there is no reason they will want to stop the action and love which they have received all day and willingly go to sleep. There are children like that, but they're usually the neighbor's kids.

So we've learned it's better to reach the end of the day with a smile and not exhausted, but what happens if both children are crying? If both stay up at night? They both want "mommy" or "daddy"...

Then what do you do? Simply stick to the instructions.

If one is asleep and the other wakes him or her up, it's not the end of the world. We will not get upset with the one who woke up the other. We will respond with the mantra: "It's night, we sleep." And if it's a baby, we touch him or her, say "Hushhh" and leave, letting him or her go back to the sleeping process. If you don't create a drama out of the situation, it will not become one. And remember: do not get upset with the child who woke up the baby. Don't say, "Shhh, you woke up your brother." Just repeat the mantra, **"Hushhh… it's night, we sleep!"**

When you are consistent, this saga will decrease every day. I promise! I remind you that you don't need to be tough with children, just consistent! Consistency pays off and is very good for the children (and for you, the parents, as well). If you have three children or more, learn to organize things in a way that will be best and most convenient for your schedules, and the principles are the same. When one of the kids particularly annoys you, ask yourself quietly if you would give him or her up. Try to answer this question only after he or she has fallen asleep.

When you start sleep training your baby, and he or she has an older sibling (3-year-old or older) who sleeps a full night, I would recommend explaining to the older child about the process you are about to go through with the baby. Of course, the explanation needs to be adjusted to the child's age and cognitive ability. I would recommend doing it through a story. Children love stories. Stories have special powers and influence. Children can relate to almost any message when it is presented in the form of a story. With a story we can relay to the child what the baby needs to go through in the process of learning to sleep.

Like in any good story, there needs to be a hero. Guess who the hero will be in the story that you tell your child? That's right, the older sibling.

I would tell the following story to the older sibling to facilitate co-operation. Of course, you can tell your own story, this is just a sample story with the hero as baby Amy's older sister whose parents are teaching her to sleep using the "Shhh… at Night We Sleep" method.

"We bought an interesting book today called "Shhh…at Night We Sleep" written by a sleep fairy. She teaches little babies like Amy how to sleep. Sleeping, as you know, is good. In the book it says that at night babies like Amy can make noises and even cry. It could take some time before we come into the room. In the meantime, Amy needs to learn from her older sister that at night we sleep! So, what does the sleep fairy ask of the big sister? Guess."

"She asks that you continue to sleep even when you hear Amy making noise. Close your eyes tightly so that Amy can also learn that at night you close your eyes and sleep! The sleep fairy says that you cannot get up because then Amy will learn that at night you get up. Can you help us with that?"

Wait for the child's response. In my experience children like to be the heroes of the story and also to help their parents. They feel of value and importance when they are asked to help, especially it makes them out to be big and strong.

I always like to have a Plan B, though. In case the child says, "I don't want to" or "I can't." It's important not to force him or her to accept your opinion. You want the child to cooperate willingly.

I suggest that you respond, "Okay, we will try to manage on our own and we hope that she does not disturb you too much."

With that, end the conversation about the little sister who is learning how to sleep. The message has been passed on. At night, when he or he she wakes up from the noise, there is a good chance that he or she will continue to sleep. If the older child gets up anyway, you know how to respond. Put him or her back in bed and say "**It's night, we sleep!**" And if he or she says that her little sister is disturbing her, repeat the mantra, "It's night, we sleep! It's night… we sleep!"

The next night, it will no longer be beneficial for the child to get up. Getting up just to hear the same mantra again and again isn't worth it. When both children will sleep in the same room you will feel a great satisfaction. It will happen sooner than you can imagine. It all depends on your determination and especially your consistency in the process.

# "Maybe"

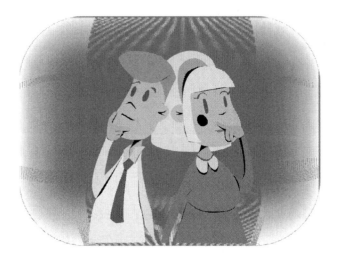

"Maybe" is a very important word in life in general, and especially in the process of raising children. But it does have its disadvantages.

On the one hand it is important because it's a word which always makes us think that there are more possibilities. It allows us to think wide as opposed to narrow, regardless of what area of life we are talking about. It is a wonderful word because every negative thought, when one adds a "maybe" to it, isn't really so bad. I use it daily. When I am upset with someone or at something I try to use the word "maybe" in my head. Maybe it's the special way in which I perceive this instance? Maybe it isn't what is really happening. Maybe....

Parents actually use "maybe" with their children in a negative way, usually with a worried look on the face.

What's the link between the word "maybe" and the "Shhh…at Night We Sleep" method? Maybe I should explain.

When you see and get a sense from your child, you find yourselves asking every once in a while if maybe something is hurting him or her. Maybe he or she needs something? Sometimes the answer is a clear yes or no, but there are many cases in which the answer is not definite and it stays in the "maybe" zone. How is this word linked to your baby's sleep? Well, a baby who has received everything he or she needs during the day should not be hurt by anything at night. A sick child shows clear signs during the day and in the hours preceding sleep time. Even the infamous colic pain, which may start at around the age of 2-weeks, ends towards the age of 3-months and can no longer be an excuse for putting the baby to sleep in your arms or with other aids.

If you feel that your baby is coming up with something, consider a doctor's visit or giving the child a pain reliever for the night. Healthy babies should not have any pains during the night, just as a healthy adult should not have any pains during the night.

Healthy adults go to sleep, and nobody picks us up or rocks us between sleep cycles because maybe something is hurting us.

Even if maybe your baby is experiencing teething discomfort, there is a solution for it: pain reliever prior to going to bed. Teeth do not start to come in specifically at night and at the moment of transition between sleep cycles. And, if "maybe" I am wrong,

give the baby a pain reliever at night. One night. Not for six months.

If you think or feel that your child is experiencing an illness or something dangerous requiring medical intervention, do not hesitate to seek medical attention. It is better to go to a doctor or to the emergency room a few times for nothing than to not get help in one critical instance. I am not referring to these cases and I trust your parental instincts, knowledge, and experience. I'm talking about cases in which we have a healthy and tired child, and you find all sorts of reasons or

192 | FROM SUNSET TO SUNRISE

excuses to pick up, rock, and nurse him or her during hours that a baby should not be doing any of those things.

There are parents who will say that maybe their baby wants love and touch during the night. To these parents I respond, "maybe," but at night we don't give love and touch because that is not what a baby needs. Parents need to do what their baby needs. At night, we need sleep. This is not a time for love. A baby does not need touch 24/7. On the contrary: a baby who gets everything that he or she needs during the day, including love and touch, is a baby who does not need love at night.

If you work late and barely get to see your baby during the day, then there are two needs that are created in you, the parents:

A need to be with the baby, because you miss him or her

A need to clear your conscience

Parents miss their children, they love them, enjoy watching them grow up and develop. Nowadays, many parents work late so they don't get to spend enough time with their children. When the baby wakes up in the middle of the night, the parents also get "quality time" with their baby, so the baby gets used to waking up at those hours because the fun is mutual. The problem is that one day, the parents discover that they are very tired. They find out that when their baby wakes up during the night he or she is not at his or her best during the day. Today's parents also read a lot of research indicating the importance of sleep to their baby's physical and mental health, and they want their baby to sleep.

Parents' guilt is also a significant contributing factor to sleeping disorders in babies. The parents feel bad that days and years pass by and they didn't get to spend enough time raising their child. These parental feelings cause them to start taking care of and loving their child during the night because they think that their baby needs love and touch. Maybe he or she misses you, maybe you miss him or her, and then the night becomes your quality time together because you feel guilty about not being at home during the day. But, what is for sure and not "maybe," is that **you both need to sleep**. You and your baby.

I suggest that you make changes to your quality time with your children. Change your baby's sleep patterns and, following that, improve your own sleep as well. Parents also list the digestive and urinary systems as excuses to wake the child up. Maybe the baby wet his or her diaper. In this case, I also advise to not change diapers during the night. As long as it does not happen often and become a habit, then it can sometimes be okay. But in general, a baby that does not nurse at night usually wakes up with a dry diaper. You would be surprised at what a young age the bladder is already strong enough to control urination. There are babies who are potty trained by the age of 12 months! If you get your child accustomed to his diaper being changed during the night then it will become a habit, and there is nothing stronger than the force of habit. Some babies have especially sensitive skin on their bottoms and in cases like this I recommend putting cream on the entire area under the diaper to minimize the contact of urine with the skin, but changing the diaper in the middle of the night on a regular basis? That isn't the proper course of action for parents who want their baby to sleep 10-12 hours nonstop at night.

If you think that maybe your baby is miserable because you are requiring him or her to fall asleep on his or her own and not in your arms, I would like to tell you that if you have a healthy child, they are not miserable. On the other hand, he or she could be miserable during the day following a night without continuous sleep, and you too would be miserable. A tired baby with tired parents is a bigger problem.

If you think that at night you would like to play because your baby is curious, aware, and does not like to sleep, I am telling you that you are wrong. Your baby really does not want or need to play at night. **Night is only for sleeping!**

Also, the baby is not afraid at night! If he or she is younger than 12 months, he or she doesn't even know that there are things from which to be afraid. If he or she is older than 12 months and is taken care of during the day, receives love and has a bond with you, then at night he or she will not be afraid!

At Night We Sleep.

If a toddler has fears and anxieties, then he or she will also display them during the day, not just at night when Mom or Dad are not able to give additional or special attention. You should know that at night your baby does not want you. Your baby expects you to help him or her sleep. If you rock or sit next to him or her at night, you are interfering with his or her sleep. You are interfering with his or her learning how to sleep a full night on his or her own. During the day, he or she wants and needs a lot from you. But, at night we sleep!

Many things in nature involve cycles. The tides and the seasons are good examples of cycles in nature. The sun's rays hit water, heat it, cause it to vaporize, the vapors go up, cool down, condense and create clouds that bring rain down and so on. Everything moves in cycles.

Day and night are also created by the turning of the earth on its axis and repeat in cycles of light and dark. As is written in the Bible:

**"And God said, 'Let there be light.' And there was light. And God saw the light that it was good, and God divided the light from the darkness. God called the light Day, and the darkness He called Night. And there was evening and there was morning, the first day."**

- *Genesis 1:3-5*

There is a time to feed, hug, kiss, play, and smile. Night is a time to sleep. That too is a part of a cycle in nature. So do not let the word "maybe" prevent your baby from sleeping a full night. Maybe he or she will not like the idea at first, but I am convinced and promise you that after three days on average you will be happier and significantly less tired.

# Implementing the Method – on a Flight

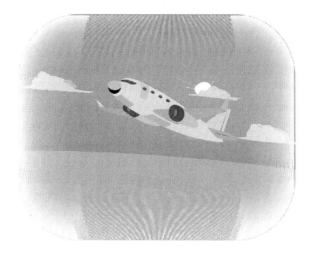

My parents used to fly on vacations without us kids. They claimed that a vacation involving flights with children costs double and is half the fun. There are parents who these days still view things this way, and when they go on vacation they trust their children to the loving hands of grandma and grandpa or another significant adult. These parents are unwilling to pay the price for breaking the routine and the discomfort for the children and themselves during the flight and vacation. It is a matter of opinion, of course, and every parent knows what is best for them and their children. There is no one correct approach. Whatever works for you. In any case, if you are one of those parents who want or need to fly with your babies and children, I want you to know that the "Shhh…at Night We Sleep" method is applicable in the air too.

When the flight is during the day (which I believe is the best time for a flight with babies and children) and the baby or child is supposed to be awake, this is wonderful. It could even be an experience. Babies and children can be occupied in creative and fun ways. It all depends on the child's age. If the baby is under the age of 18 months, there is a chance that he or she may need a short nap during the flight, even if it is a day flight. If the child is over 2 years old , you should bring a toy, coloring book, or a story book. Sometimes a familiar book or toy will do the job and sometimes it will be a new book or toy which will occupy him or her sitting quietly during the flight. Either way, a flight is not yours or your baby's natural surroundings. Usually I like to start from the positive aspect of what I want to discuss or write about, but this time I will start with what a plane does not have that is required for good sleep:

- No room or bed
- No quiet
- No darkness
- No comfort

And while I'm on the subject of what is lacking, then I will continue with what not to do when your baby needs to sleep while you are on a plane.

Do not nurse or feed the baby when he or she doesn't need it. It will only burden the stomach and cause discomfort and he or she will not sleep as well, if at all.

Do not talk to him or her and try to calm him or her down with words or when he or she needs to sleep.

Do not rock him or her and keep changing positions. It hinders the falling asleep process.

Do not occupy him or her with toys or stimuli which might raise adrenaline levels, which are already higher than normal in this situation.

Sometimes you need to take a night flight, and then you don't have a choice. You have to wake the baby up to get to the airport. At the beginning, it's actually rather nice, he or she could even smile at you, but as time goes by and you get on the flight, tiredness overcomes the smiles and the baby starts moving restlessly in your arms, fussing and even crying.

When I am on a flight and see parents pacing up and down the aisle with their babies in their arms I want to say: "Sit down, there is no need to walk around. Sit in your seat, hug the baby, hold him or her, and don't move. Just repeat the mantra "Shhhhhh, "Shhhhhh, Shhhhhh." The baby might get annoyed at hearing the mantra in the beginning, but if you don't move and continue to hug the child and repeat it, you might be surprised how within 15 minutes (more or less, usually less) he or she will close his or her eyes and sleep. Very quickly the child will have no benefit to staying awake and will realize that he or she become calmer and his or her sleep will not be disturbed. The plane noises will quickly turn into white noise and the baby will just… sleep!

Our body moves during sleep as well. He or she will try to move occasionally and so will you. Don't worry. When the baby moves, quietly say, "Shhhhh," change his or her position and repeat the mantra if he or she wakes up.

If you usually sing him or her a lullaby before bedtime, you can sing it on the plane a few times. As long as the principle and the mantra repeat themselves, there is a chance for a smooth transition into the sleep process. In order to facilitate the process, it would be very helpful if you could put him or her in a car seat or a crib. For that purpose, you should find out if it's possible to take the car safety seat with you and put it on the plane seat. It might, on most airlines, mean paying for an additional seat, but it is much safer and the baby might sleep on it more comfortably and longer. To use the car seat, you need to make sure that it is approved for use on planes. On most airplanes the chair needs to be about 16" wide. You should check with your airline if they could supply you with a safety seat if you cannot bring your own. It is important on any flight, but especially on transAtlantic flights.

There are a few airlines who will supply a crib for babies up until the age of 9 months. The rules and regulations do vary so it's best to find out before the flight. You might also try to be seated next to a vacant seat if the flight isn't full. If you are not allowed to bring your safety seat and you don't want to chance it with a place for the baby, you can always purchase another seat next to you and improvise a bed. It's never a cheap option, but if you are taking a very long flight with the baby you might want to consider it. You can also ask to sit in the first row, and then there is usually room on the floor to lay out a heavy blanket and improvise a bed to lay the baby on.

During one of my long flights from Israel to Los Angeles, after listening to an 8-month-old baby crying in her father's arms for two hours straight as he paced along the aisle, I walked up to him and said, "Let's stand here on the side for a moment. I would like to suggest something." By the look on his face I could tell that he thought that I wanted to complain about the crying. I put his mind at ease and told him that I was a sleep coach. I asked that he hold his baby cradled in his arms horizontally and not vertically on his chest. The baby resisted and I told him to keep her in this position and just say to her: "Shhhhh." And I did the same. "Shhhhh." I promised I'll soon explain to him what I was striving for, but until then that he shouldn't move her and not allow her to get out of his embrace. Within ten minutes she fell asleep as her body lay relaxed in her father's arms and he sat down in his seat. I stood next to him and explained that it was those attempts at calming her in all sorts of inconsistent ways that was preventing the baby from going into a sleep process in a noisy and uncomfortable airplane.

As for food, I recommend keeping the same meal routine as much as possible. Nursing babies need to be nursed according to the routine. For older children, you can order a child's meal.

Things to do before flying with children:

- Always find out if the flight is leaving on time. You should not wander around with children for hours at the airport.
- It is always best to have the baby sit next to a window or next to a person and not in the aisle, the most difficult place to fall asleep on a plane.
- Start putting your baby to sleep as soon as he or she seems tired. You don't have to wait for the plane to take off. Even though people will be standing and wandering around you, putting their bags in the overhead bins, if you act in accordance with the method, the noise and interest around will all turn into white noise. However, if you are flying with a 24- months-or-older child, I recommend waiting until after takeoff.

What you should bring with you to the flight:

- Bottles and formula for nursing babies (breastfeeding moms have one less thing to worry about)
- A teddy bear or a familiar object
- Eardrops to help in case of strong ear pressure during takeoff or landing
- Baby/child's blanket
- Pillow, which you could put on your legs for the baby to sleep on

- Eye masks for babies and children – some may show signs of discomfort when they are put on, but within a few minutes they may fall into a good sleep thanks to the lack of exposure to light

**Did you know?**

*During takeoff and landing it's advisable to nurse your baby (if he or she is nursing) or give a bottle with a little bit of water, while older children are advised to chew gum, like adults, to avoid ear pressure.*

# Flying on Vacation – Who wants to come?

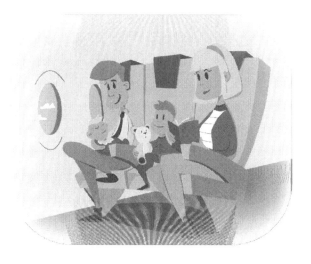

I hope that you're all excited about going on a vacation, or maybe you have just returned from one. Either way, it's time to pay the price and there is a chance that you are suffering from jet lag. Jet lag describes the situation in which your biological clock hasn't yet adjusted itself to the new time zone. It usually takes a few days of dizziness and being tired until the levels of light reorder your biological clock.

There are a few things you can do to overcome this situation:

Adults can start changing their biological clock towards the time at the destination a few minutes every day about a week before the flight. Don't change anything in the babies and children's schedule in the days before the flight.

Find the flight which best fits your schedule and allows you to sleep on the flight while it is nighttime at the destination. This applies to the parents as well as babies and children. If you are traveling east it is best to fly out early in the day and if you are traveling west, fly out late.

When you get on the plane set your watches to the destination's new time zone. If it's nighttime at the destination, close your eyes (best to use an eye mask) and go to sleep. If it's morning or noontime, stay awake and eat your meals accordingly. Light is very important for synchronizing your internal clock, but so is food. Research shows that if you have jet lag and eat indiscriminately , it may take up to a week to get over the jet lag, but when you limit food and organize your meals according to the new time zone you can overcome jet lag faster. The best advice that I can give you in this matter is not to eat prior to the flight and, when you get to the destination, eat the first meal local time. Babies and children are best kept quietly occupied, not aroused. If it's a young baby, sing him or her a lullaby a few times. There is a chance that the constant repetitiveness will put the baby to sleep. Babies and children should also have their meal times organized as quickly as possible. The more in sync they are with the destination's time the quicker they will get over the change in the internal clock.

If after arrival the children cannot stay awake and want to sleep in the middle of the day at the destination, you should let them, but it is best to wake them up for a while after an hour and a half.

If you return from the east in the morning or before noon try to keep your children awake until the latest they can hold up to match evening time, which is earlier relative to the east coast. Thus if they already look tired at 3 PM, try to hold them up until 7 PM. The next day, don't wake them up but open the windows in the morning and invite the sunlight into their room. Make a normal amount of noise as opposed to keeping quiet, and they will slowly wake up. During the day allow them a nap appropriate for their age, and at night put them down an hour later than the previous night, and so on until you reach the original bedtime.

If the baby or child wakes up in the middle of the night stay with him or her around his or her bed and try to get him or her back to sleep according to the instructions of the method. Do not start feeding at night.

If you are planning a family trip with kids older than 2 (and under 12), you should tell them about the flight only at the day of the flight and not the night or days before because they could lose sleep out of excitement.

# Vacation and Sleep – It's Not a Problem

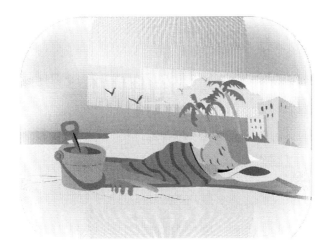

According to Dictionary.com, a vacation is defined as an extended period of recreation, especially one spent away from home or in traveling.

And, free is defined as not under the control or in the power of another; able to act or do as one wishes.

So the next time you want to go with your children on a vacation, define first what it is that you mean. Will this be a break from work? Will you really have the freedom to decide what to do at any moment?

Many parents tell me that they went on a vacation with their baby and children and that it was anything but a vacation. I also know many parents who love to travel around the country and around the world with their children and come back feeling that it was a great experience for all. And yet, when it comes to sleep there is a theoretical problem. The baby or child is in a different place than he or she is used to. The room, the bed, the people sleeping in the same room, the atmosphere, the sounds, and even the smells are all different. There are babies and children who will have a hard time getting used to this change and the process of going to sleep will take longer than usual, with spells of waking up and difficulty to go back to sleep. However, I can tell you that it's pretty easy to keep the wonderful sleeping habits that you had at home.

There is no real reason for lack of sleep during your vacation. Here is what you should do for that:

First of all, stick to the method's guidelines when on vacation. But remember that on vacations it becomes easier to break the routine and that has a price. You break it, you pay for it!

Try to keep the regular bedtime as much as possible, as well as lowering activity about half an hour beforehand.

If the children are ages 2 years and up, they should be made a part of the responsibility for the process. "You are responsible for telling everyone what time it is," "You are responsible for collecting the toys," etc. (age appropriate, of course).

If you have decided to completely break the rules until the children just drop to sleep on the floor, that's okay too. Just don't break any rules in the middle of the night. No food and water, just the mantra.

Don't be upset with the children, because they didn't initiate the vacation and it isn't their responsibility to keep their sleeping habits. It's the sole responsibility of the parents.

Don't fight with them over food. Some parents will demand that the children eat right now because "we are not at home and there won't be any food later." If there won't be, they will learn the next day to sit down and eat: "Too bad you didn't sit down with us and eat, there was plenty of food. Tomorrow in the morning the dining room will reopen." No child will starve to death if for one evening he or she does not eat "enough."

When you return home, you start over with no anger. Understand that the children also will have a hard time getting back into the routine. After an average of three days you should be back to continuous good sleep.

Bring things and toys with you that the baby is used to and are related to the sleeping ceremony, as well as his or her personal blanket.

Parents tend to make a mistake of getting mad at children when they "misbehave" and threaten that it will be the last family vacation. But:

It won't hold water, so no use threatening them.

It will ruin the atmosphere and the vacation for you and them. Take a deep breath before you speak.

When there's tension between the children draw their attention with a game, a conversation or talk about your next destination.

Relieve the tension with something helpful and positive.

# A New Baby in the Family

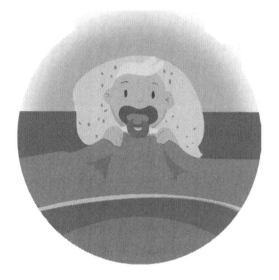

Congratulations, you have a new baby!

As a certified nurse, I was educated not just to treat current problems, but also to think about how best to prevent them from happening. There is research evidence that sleeping problems can be prevented as early as the pregnancy stage.

During the first few days after birth the baby will spend most of the time sleeping. But very quickly he or she will become addicted to one or more of life's pleasures. The most common ones are the breast, the pacifier, the bottle, the rocking, white noise, and more. Parents, like children, are very creative and will try anything, and I mean anything to get the baby to sleep quickly. Here are 8 good habits to teach the little ones to sleep between meals. Before I list them I would like to emphasize this: Breastfeeding babies about 8 sessions a day. It is important to start feeding during the day as soon as the baby starts moving in bed (as crying is a later sign of hunger) so that most sessions are during the day and less during the night, but still the baby needs to be breastfed at night as needed.

When the baby needs to sleep (whether it is day or night) he or she must be provided with unchanging sleeping conditions that may help him or her in the process of falling asleep, such as a dark room and less distractions such as noise, games and screens.

Do not place the baby in bed without checking his or her hunger level. A hungry baby will not sleep well.

Create a consistent ceremony.

"Teddy bear goes to sleep, doggy goes to sleep, dolly goes to sleep, and Sally goes to sleep." During the first days it will seem strange to take the baby in your arms and say goodbye to toys that he or doesn't even know yet.

Do not put the baby to sleep in your arms or use any external aid. He or she should be put in bed while still awake.

Make sure the baby's room temperature is at 70-74°F, and that the environment is clean and well-ventilated.

A baby who sleeps well during the day will sleep better during the night, so make sure he or she sleeps during the day.

Respond to the baby in the same manner every time that he or she has a hard time falling asleep. Consistency is the cornerstone of good habit formation.

Avoid reacting too quickly to every cry from the baby during the sleeping process. Wait a minute before you respond. During this minute the baby could go back to sleep without you interrupting the process.

# Being an Excellent Parent is Dangerous

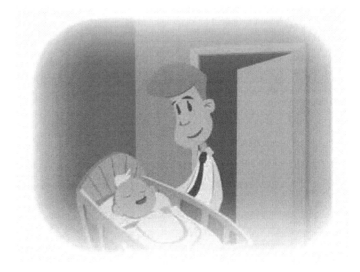

Any experienced parent knows that no matter how much we strive to be excellent parents, we will always make mistakes. Why? Because to err is human, and we learn from mistakes. I see excellent parents in my clinic, who only want the best for their children. When parents realize that if they'll be very good parents their children will happier and content, the parents are on the right path. Parents who don't set themselves unrealistic expectations to be perfect parents are those who make fewer mistakes; they know to stop every once in a while, think about what is right for them and their children, improve and fix what is required.

Raising children and giving them what they need is work. Hard work. The good thing is that it is accompanied by a lot of pleasure and satisfaction. I'm for good work, not hard work. I always tell my children: "Don't work hard, work well!" This means not feeling obligated to be an excellent parent. Being an excellent parent is dangerous. What is excellent for one child may not be the right thing for another child in the same family.

In my entire career I've never met parents who could be very good parents without eating properly, sleeping well, and being frustrated with daily life. There were some about whom I could say, "Wow, these parents are excellent," but I soon discovered that their problems were popping up in other places: their relationship, at work, or with friends. They invested all of their energy in their children, and unjustifiably so. Children shouldn't need all your energy. They need to get what they need. Usually, you would be surprised, they don't need much. Those who are in constant need are usually the ones whose parents thought they needed a lot of everything and created the habit themselves.

I love the current generation of parents — wise and sophisticated. This generation invents things, improves technology and the quality of life. Yet the generation growing up these days is one that does not settle for "very good." When their lives are good, it's not enough for them. Everything has to be excellent. And they adopt this attitude to parenting too. I know that I am generalizing here. Those who aren't like that, great! I am talking about the majority because the majority rules. Parents want to be excellent at parenting. Nothing less!

The strive for excellence in parenting is the enemy. It is an unrealistic aspiration which causes a lot of stress and leads to couples fighting if one person insists that the other be an excellent parent, too, according to their view of excellence, of course. The moment the "excellent" parent experiences failure, his or her mood is affected, sometimes significantly, to the point that it may affect his functioning. People who view excellence as a basic condition for a sense of belonging are people who are doomed to fail in regards to their emotional condition. This is a pattern that they often bring to parenting. He gets frustrated when he fails to reach his standards. An excellent parent is one who is constantly in competition, with a spouse, other parents, or with the extended family. While you struggle to be excellent (especially compared to others), you are wasting valuable time. Don't waste your lives in competing with someone else. Be the best that you can be and not by way of comparison to others. That is the difference between an achieving person and a competitive person. To be an achiever is good. It brings forth the best version of ourselves for our children, our family, and others. To be competitive is a waste of valuable time and especially energy, which is of limited supply in our lives. Parents who strive to be excellent parents are usually in great stress, from fear of not holding up to expectations set by themselves or others.

One of the mistakes excellent parents make is setting boundaries, which is particularly hard on them. Setting boundaries is not exactly the experience that the excellent parent has dreamed about in his or her relationship with his or her child. "If I was so excellent, then why is he reacting to me this way?" Setting a boundary is an unpleasant moment for both parties. The child may feel that the parent doesn't understand him or her and is not being good to him or her. If you are now saying to yourselves, "Oh, I am an excellent parent who sets boundaries when it's necessary," then you are not excellent parents but very good parents. In my opinion, that is a wonderful thing.

When a parent settles for "very good" and knows how to be grateful for what he or she has, he or she is usually happier and more optimistic, which is a reflection of his or her relationship with him- or herself and with his or her children.

It's the same with sleep. During the day, when the excellent parent does everything that he or she should, and at night the baby cries because he or she does not want to fall asleep on his or her own, then the excellent parent will not put him or her in bed and expect him or her to put him- or herself to sleep. The excellent parent will expect that he or she has to assist the baby, because that is what an excellent parent does.

Be good parents, and provide your child with everything that he or she needs. It is important that children grow up with the sense that they have not just a physical place but also a place in people's hearts, especially when it comes to their parents, who are the pillars in their lives. Sometimes children need to be taught certain things: to build, to play, to deal with failures or losses. Teach them.

In his book "Children: The Challenge," Driekurs, who was Adler's student and successor, writes that parents need to invest time in coaching and teaching children life skills. Sometimes children need education and boundaries, and other times they need to be taught the limits of what is allowed and what is possible. Sometimes children need to sleep, and then they need to be taught the skills of falling asleep. Yes, falling asleep is a skill which a good parent needs to teach.

And one other thing. Excellent parents don't sleep, because some of them strive for excellence in other aspects of life as well. They tend to give up on sleep in favor of achievement and competitiveness, which comes at the expense of sleep. Being excellent can be dangerous!

**"A time to embrace, and a time to refrain from embracing…"**

*- Ecclesiastes 3:5*

# Managing Daylight Savings Time

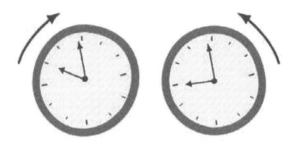

## Daylight Saving Time: Spring Forward

Two days a year, every year, I answer the most phone calls. A day before the changing of the clock to daylight savings time, and a day before it's moved back. People don't like changes. Even those who declare that they are spontaneous and proponents of change and challenges ultimately prefer the familiar. The thought of changing the child's sleeping habits causes discomfort to many parents.

On the day the clock changes for daylight savings time in the fall, we lose light hours in the afternoon but gain an hour of sleep (which is why this is my favorite time change), and in the spring we gain hours of light in the evening, but lose an hour of sleep when changing the clock.

Babies and children will respond differently to the changing time of spring and fall. The better the child's sleeping habits, the quicker he or she might adapt to the change.

It can take adults two to three days to adjust to the change, while for babies and children it could take up to 7-10 days. Parents who were used to waking up with their baby at 6 AM suddenly find themselves with a baby in their hand at 5 AM. It isn't fun, but if you're patient within a week your may get used to the new clock and return to his regular wake up time. You only need patience.

Here are a few pointers to shorten the process of adapting to the change:

Don't stray from the baby or child's daily schedule which he or she was used to.

Gradually move the bedtime ten minutes every day until you reach the desired time again. There may be days when bedtime happens while there's still light outside. It is advisable to darken the house using heavy drapes or shutters in order to create artificial darkness.

Remember that babies and children may become restless during periods of change to their bedtime and waking schedules. Be patient. It all falls back into place after a few days.

## Daylight Saving Time: Fall Back

I particularly like when we move the time one hour back at fall and we get another hour of sleep. Some children might wake up too early, when they're used to waking up.

How can we help them handle this change?

Some claim that it's advisable to put the children to bed according to fall time a few days before the change. I believe you should wait for the day you change the time. Either way it will take them a few days to adjust, so why put you and them through it before the actual time change?

I recommend pushing back bedtime by about five minutes every evening. It isn't a significant change per day and it may assist in the adjustment.

When the baby wakes up early in the morning , don't take him or her out of bed but wait until he or she starts complaining. When that happens, go to him or her, caress him or her, and leave for up to ten minutes before eventually taking him or her out of bed. The idea is to give the child a chance to see you and go back to sleep. If he or she doesn't go back to sleep – take him or her out of bed.

The baby should be put to bed at the same hour, in the spring and fall.

In any case where a baby or child presents difficulty, you should sit next to him or her and continue to caress and calm him or her down for two to three days. No longer than that, as it may cause dependency and habit.

Babies and children may exhibit restlessness at the changes in the transition between sleep and waking. Be patient. It will get back to normal within a few days.

Older children need to be explained about the change and its purpose. Children like to be included and this way you will gain their cooperation as well.

It isn't advisable to complain next to the children, but rather state that this is a given and we all have to get used to it. This is how we teach children that there are situations in life that you need to get used to.

**"I will form good habits and become their slave. And how will I accomplish this difficult feat? Through these scrolls it will be done, for each scroll contains a principle which will drive a bad habit from my life and replace it with one which will bring me closer to success."**

- *Og Mandino*

# Old Wives' Tales

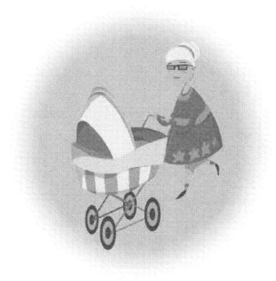

Behind every baby there is a grandmother. Well, okay, a grandfather too. With that, and with all due respect, the grandmothers enjoy giving constant advice.

If I could give young parents one piece of advice, it would be, "listen to grandmother's advice."

They are usually golden nuggets, derived from years of life and child-rearing experience. You don't have to take every piece of advice, but I do recommend listening to it.

There are cases in which you would want or need to live with your parents (the baby's grandparents). When you decide to teach your baby to sleep a full night utilizing the "Shhh…at Night We Sleep" method, you will need to explain to grandma and grandpa that you are starting a process of teaching your babies how to sleep. It may seem strange to some of the grandparents.

They might say, "What? You were not taught how to sleep by sleep coaches or trainers and you slept wonderfully at night."

Others might say, "Wow, how wonderful it is that there are people to help these days with teaching your baby how to sleep, because in our day we didn't know what sleep was."

Either way, if you want your parents' help, I suggest that you let them read this book. They may show an understanding of the process and help you. I think that if you are living with them it is important to include them. It will be considerate of you. Ultimately, the decision to start teaching how to sleep is yours.

And to you, dear **grandparents**, circumstances brought your children (and grandchildren) to live with you. I am sure that it is great, and yet there are times when it isn't easy. Sleep is a basic need and in its absence, the household members are less patient, more prone to lose their temper and make demands, and that is not a desirable situation. Please respect your children's decision to go with their baby through the process of teaching him or her sleeping skills, even if it is not what you did in the past.

In my experience, at the end of the process you might admit that "it's too bad that they didn't do this earlier" (a quote from a letter by Grandma Rose).

The greatest help you can provide will be allowing them to follow the instructions diligently and encouraging them.

If the couple decides to go to a clinic for consultation, I have no doubt that you will be happily received as role partners.

# Sleep Training Vs Sleep Counseling

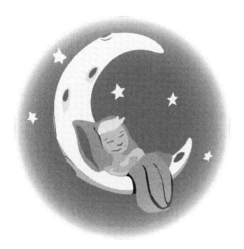

Sleep counseling or sleep training? Who should we turn to? Turns out that many parents really don't know where to turn and who might be able to solve the sleeping problems of their babies and children.

What is sleep training and what is sleep counseling? In the "Shhh… at Night We Sleep" method, our team of counselors work with the coaching approach.

Coaching and training are two therapeutic platforms that are meant to help the baby create good sleeping habits. They are not the same, and each can help in a different way. They have some aspects in common and some differences. One of the most significant differences is that in counseling, the knowledge is the counselor's, and with coaching the knowledge is with the coached.

While the baby does not pick up the phone to schedule a session to deal with his sleeping issues, he or she is most certainly the one going through the process and the knowledge of how to fall asleep on his or her own is his or hers alone. Since this process is performed via the parents, in our method we combine principles of coaching and advising.

## Sleep Training

Personal coaching deals with the set of values, opinions, and attitudes of a person towards him-or herself and towards the world, and is measured by its results. It could be one of the most important experiences that a person goes through during his or her lifetime. The coaching helps a person reach insights, encourages him or her to be more effective, puts him or her in touch with his or her goals, and helps fulfill those goals.

The purpose of personal training is to minimize the distance between the desired and the reality, with focused work for a limited time. Coaching has a very well defined goal. The coach is a partner and encourager of the person being coached. Coaching is based on learning, thinking, and acting. The coach-coachee relationship is mutual. While the doing and the success belong to the coachee, they are achieved through the coach's ability to assist, encourage, and listen.

The coachee commits to the process, to learning and assimilating what is taught, and practicing the acquired insights through the coaching process.

The coach is committed to sharing his or her knowledge, provide feedback, and encourage the coachee to assimilate and maintain the behavioral changes.

Coaching as a platform that promotes achieving goals is actually derived from the field of sports. The coaching view in sports maintains that the success of the process depends on the players or the team, as well as on the coach.

The same goes with sleep coaching. When parents believe that their baby should sleep and they set before them this noble cause, they can work towards their vision assisted by a sleep coach who works with them on achieving their goals and defining a precise time table.

In my experience babies between 3-24-months-old can learn to fall asleep on their own within three days on average. Ages 2 and up – within five days on average.

The parents commit to the process and the sleep coach commits to supporting, encouraging, and helping. It's the parents' success, with a certain portion from the coach. Both sides have to take responsibility on their part.

Personal coaching has been shown to be the most effective way of fulfilling one's personal potential and of improving personal and professional performance in all aspects of life, including sleep. People usually welcome change when they are rewarded for their efforts. Thus, following sleep coaching, when the baby sleeps a full night, the parents and the baby are rewarded by quality continuous sleep with all its advantages.

## Sleep Counseling

Counseling is based on expertise and knowledge. The counselor is a professional with experience in a particular field who passes his knowledge on to his client. A business coach, for example, can tell his client that he is not marketing his business efficiently and correctly. A nutritionist can tell her clients that they aren't eating right. In sleep counseling, the parents will be told what they are doing wrong, and what to improve or change in order to create better sleeping habits for the baby. When the parents come to a sleep counselor, she will ask questions about the habits of the babies, tell the parents what she believes they are doing incorrectly, and provide them with her knowledge and experience in order to solve their sleeping issue. The consultant provides his knowledge to the patient.

Sometimes when a couple comes in for sleep counseling, they're advised to seek a pediatrician for a referral to a sleep lab. In such rare cases, there is no need for sleep coaching, at least not until it has been established that the problem is not organic.

With the "Shhh...at Night We Sleep" method, the sleep coaches have the knowledge and experience, and the entire process is centered on the principal goal: teaching the baby to sleep through utilization of the internal endogenic motion, which in my method is referred to as the Transitional Motion. The knowledge and the ability are innately possessed by the baby, and the sleep coach can help the baby achieve the goal of continuous sleep with the assistance of the parents.

# When the Baby is Already Sleeping and You Aren't

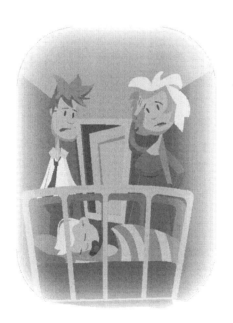

Many parents tell me that after they have taught their baby to sleep, they find themselves with a sleeping baby while they themselves are left awake. The beacon of light is that even in these cases, there is something that can be done.

It's important that you don't worry, especially if you had not had chronic sleeping disorders before. It's probably secondary insomnia, which very likely has been caused by the interruptions to your biological clock from the need to adjust to the baby's sleeping and waking schedule.

Now that your baby has learned how to sleep, you need to go back and get used to your original biological clock.

This kind of insomnia usually disappears with the person's adjustment to the change which he or she is experiencing, and thus there is no special reason for medical or behavioral treatment but rather implementing this advice:

Go to sleep as close to the baby's bedtime as possible. While it may sound unrealistic, with an open mind and moving away from the comfort zone of your habits you will see that it is entirely possible. You need to remember that if you put the baby to bed at 6 PM and he or she sleeps (a good) 11 hours, he or she will wake up at 5 AM, which is a very early time for you. I don't really expect you to turn in at 6 PM, but the general idea is to push forward your bedtime by about one or two hours, and then five in the morning will not seem so outlandish.

We are all familiar with the term "hygiene," which usually refers to bodily cleanliness. In the sleep field there is a term called sleep hygiene.

**How do you practice sleep hygiene?**
Make sure you keep a clean and proper sleep environment, clean of interruptions.

Make sure you have a comfortable bed and mattress, pleasant room temperature, and a dark room which minimizes noises.

Keep the bed as a place for sleep and intimacy only. There should be no screens in the place of sleep! Why is that important? Because you should be conditioned to the fact that when you get into bed, it's for sleeping. And then you and your brain will be clear that it's now sleep time and not time for working, surfing the net, or dealing with today's issues. Some people like to fall asleep watching TV. If you're addicted to watching movies, take the TV out of the bedroom.

Avoid coffee and any other drink containing caffeine such as cola, hot chocolate, energy drinks, and chocolate because caffeine is an arousing substance that stimulates the central nervous system and is also known to be a diuretic. Yet there are people who report that a cup of coffee before bedtime actually helps them fall asleep or does not hinder their sleep or its quality. I am such a person, able to sleep with or without coffee.

Make sure you go to bed and wake up at the same time every day. Keeping a routine of waking and sleeping helps keep the hormonal cycles balanced and the biological clock regular. Even after a sleepless night avoid sleeping during the day, and turn in only at night.

Eat an early light dinner. The digestion of a heavy meal might hinder the quality of sleep as well as cause heartburn. Hunger can also get in the way of falling asleep, so if you feel hunger before falling asleep you can add a snack or a fruit.

Leave all your worries outside the room. How do you do that? During the early evening hours write on a piece of paper all the tasks for the following day, and if there are things which are worrying you beyond these tasks then it's a good idea to write them too. Don't worry, all the problems and worries will wait for you tomorrow. No fairies or angels will be coming around to set them all straight, but if you sleep well, there is a better chance that you can solve them in the morning.

Take the clock out of the room (my recommendation). In a house with babies there is a chance that you may not need an alarm clock, but if you don't have a choice because you need one, then place it away from you or cover it with a little towel, so that you don't see what time it is from your bed. Following the clock every time that you wake up only increases stress and worry. "What, it's already two o'clock in the morning and I have not slept at all?"

Don't try to force falling asleep. If you feel that it's been 20-30 minutes and you still haven't fallen asleep, get out of bed and get back in only when you feel the need to sleep.

Exercise during the day, in the morning or afternoon. Physical activity is very important for your health, but it's important that it isn't around the time of sleep because that increases the level of arousal.

During the morning hours expose yourself to natural light. Going out with the baby for a stroll during these hours is a wonderful activity for both of you.

---

### Did you know?

*The origin of the word "hygiene" is the name of the goddess of health, Hygieia. The meaning of the name in Greek mythology is keeping clean in the bodily sense, and today we speak of sleep hygiene in the same sense.*

# Ugh! Regression

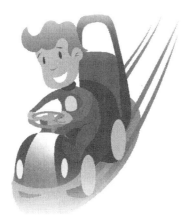

"A sorrow shared is a fool's comfort," or maybe "half a comfort."

All babies who have learned how to sleep a full night can experience regression. Sometimes it just happens for no reason, and sometimes it's a result of a tuxedo event or something that we will not be able to pinpoint. Regression doesn't occur just in babies and children, it can also occur in parents, who sometimes react differently than instructed to a change in the baby's behavior, and sometimes for no particular reason.

Parents often ask how it happened that their independentlysleeping baby has been sleeping a full night for a week now, and suddenly tonight, of all nights, he woke up twice!

There are many reasons for regression in the sleep process of babies and children, some of them overt and some covert. Sometimes it's a growth spurt, which manifests itself also in sleep. Sometimes the reason is the changing of seasons, events that happened during the day, teething, or just that he or she misses you. The most important thing to remember when regression comes knocking is to act according to the principles of the method and not to break the rules.

You broke it – You bought it!

If during an entire week there is one night that goes wrong, that's okay, as long as you remain consistent and determined. If there are a few nights a week that you call "regression", then that isn't the baby's regression, that is a regression in your response to normal waking of the baby for reasons that I have listed above. Every time you respond to the baby or the child in a manner inconsistent with the system, you might have a regression that could become a new method named after you!

# Sometimes You Need Help

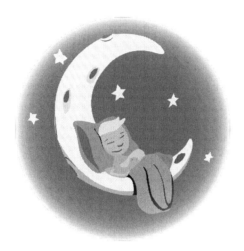

Parents who are dealing with their baby's sleeping problems and have tried everything find it hard to believe that the problem is solvable. The difficulty comes from the feeling that their case is especially hard or that their baby is particularly stubborn. In some cases, parents feel like failures because they were not successful where other parents have succeeded. In other cases, the lack of faith in a solution prevents the parents from understanding that they can get help.

There are families in which the roles of the parents are such that one is the breadwinner and the other is responsible for child rearing. When this is the case, the process of teaching the baby how to sleep independently is usually performed by one parent. This is certainly possible. I believe that every parent can and should be able to teach

230 | From Sunset to Sunrise

their baby to sleep. Yet sometimes we need help. Maybe all you need is a little encouragement and support that what you are doing is the right thing to do, or encouragement to remain consistent. In a family in which both parents share responsibilities, usually one encourages the other and reminds the other of the instructions if forgotten, and the parents work as a unified team towards the goal.

I recommend both spouses read this book because that way you will both speak the same language and can help each other succeed in your mission. If the person you have chosen for help in this process is a grandparent or a nanny, let him or her read the book too. Those working according to the "Shhh…at Night We Sleep" method need to understand the rationale for and the explanation of the steps of the method.

When you leave the baby with his or her grandparents or a babysitter and they have not read about the method, let them put the baby to sleep however they want or are used to. I promise that your baby's sleep will not be ruined. Only what the parents do is important. At a very early age babies and children can already identify who is taking care of them and how they should act in each instance. Most nights you are the ones responsible for putting your baby to sleep, and the majority rules.

If after you have read the book and followed the instructions precisely you still need guidance and assistance, the next step is to reach out to a sleep coach who works according to the "Shhh… at Night We Sleep" method.

# Questions and Answers

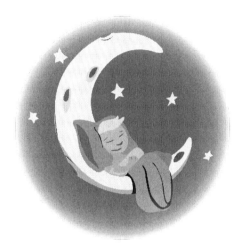

**Q:** We are a divorced couple living in two separate homes with joint custody. Is it possible to implement the method when it is followed only in one of the homes?

**A:** Of course it's possible. Babies and children learn very quickly that in one home things are done a certain way and in the other, another way. So as long as each household remains consistent, the children are less confused.

**Q:** I am in a Facebook group which contains a lot of criticism regarding sleep counseling and coaching for babies. I am concerned that sleep training might hurt the health of our baby, despite the fact that we don't sleep enough. What do you think?

**A:** There is no proof or research to show that educating babies to sleep a full night can cause the baby health problems. The discussion among different groups, especially on social media, is emotional and not at all rational. All research done on the issue of sleep training for babies indicates that it is a safe process.

**Q:** I've heard about the "Shhh…at Night We Sleep" method and it all makes sense, but I have a very hard time hearing my baby cry during the process, although he cries a lot during the day and night unrelated to the method. What should I do?

**A:** I think that your question contains the best and most correct answer: your baby cries because he is tired, sick or has a low threshold for frustration. On the contrary, after he has learned to sleep with the "Shhh…at Night We Sleep" method he will cry a lot less because he will be a more relaxed, happy, and healthy baby. My suggestion to you is that when he cries during the process (which is short, compared to other methods), think not just about what you want to hear now (a baby that isn't crying), think about what you want more than anything. I'm sure your answer will be that he sleeps a full night and enjoys all of the benefits of continuous sleep, i.e. happiness, health, happier parents, and more.

**Q:** My child is 4.5 years old and is having behavioral issues at daycare. Is it possible that this is related to the fact that he refuses to go to sleep and falls asleep only at 10:30 PM?

**A:** You didn't mention when he wakes up in the morning and whether you need to wake him up or he wakes up on his own, but it is certainly possible that a child with a sleep disturbance or sleep deprivation will develop behavioral issues because these children are usually very irritable, lack patience, and have attention difficulties.

**Q:** Do all babies succeed with sleep training?

**A:** All babies can succeed with the sleep training of this method, but there is a (small) number of parents who do not follow the instructions to the letter, parents who are not committed to the entire process. Parents who do not like to do things that they are not used to doing, even though in order to achieve results one must do something that he or she has not done yet. We can tell parents right from the first phone call when the method isn't suitable for them.

**Q:** How long will it take for our baby to sleep a full night with the "Shhh…at Night We Sleep" method?

**A:** When you act with 100% precision, your baby will sleep a full night of 10-12 hours within 3-6 days.

**Q:** Our baby is very curious and restless most of the time. From the day he was born he does not like to sleep and he keeps turning around, wanting to see everything around him. Is it possible that there are babies who are curious and don't like to sleep so that they don't miss out on anything?

**A:** All healthy babies are born curious creatures. Everything is new to them. Restlessness usually is expressed due to lack of sleep. It is a psychomotor restlessness. Tiredness in children may sometimes be expressed in over-activity rather than calming down.

**Q:** We think our 5-year-old daughter suffers from attention disorders. Ever since she was a baby she has not slept a full night. Is there a link between the two?

**A:** ADHD has been found to be statistically linked to sleeping disorders. In addition, sleep deprivation and tiredness cause symptoms which simulate attention disorders.

**Q:** Our baby was born with a sensory regulation disorder. She cannot fall asleep on her own. Is her issue with falling asleep on her own related to her sensory regulation issue?

**A:** Many babies don't know how to fall asleep mostly because of bad habits from infancy. Yet babies with oversensitivity to stimuli and deficiencies in sensory regulation have a particularly hard time transitioning from day into night. In order to get into the process, the baby needs to detach from the outside environment. A baby with oversensitivity to environmental stimuli will have a hard time detaching and getting into the sleep process.

**Q:** Will my baby's sleeping problem not just go away on its own, without treatment, when he grows up?

**A:** Regrettably, experience has shown that babies who did not learn how to sleep as infants may have sleeping issues as adults as well. It is easier to treat sleeping issues in infancy rather than in adulthood.

**Q:** I have no problem waking up two to three times a night, but during the day my baby girl does not sleep at all. Is it possible to treat only day sleep?

**A:** You may not mind waking up two to three times a night to calm your daughter down but this book is mainly about treating sleeping problems in order to avoid health issues, which happen due to sleep deprivation. In addition, day sleep is affected by night sleep. Babies who sleep well at night also sleep better during the day, and vice versa.

**Q:** My son is 4.5 months old and I was wondering if maybe I should wait until he is 12 months old and then start teaching him how to sleep.

**A:** Your son could have already been sleeping a full night for the past month and a half. Sleep is a basic need and it is very undesirable to postpone teaching your baby to sleep a full night, certainly not to wait until the age of 12 months. However, the parents decide when they're ready to start the process.

**Q:** I have 5-year-old twins and we have meat for supper before bedtime (a dairy based lunch). Could that be the reason that they are not sleeping well?

**A:** I find it hard to believe that meat for supper is the reason for your children's sleep disorders. I don't have information as to when these problems started. In regards to the nutrition only, the foods which are advisable to avoid before bedtime are sugars, legumes and meat. If you have meat for supper, try and do so at least 90 minutes before going to sleep.

**Q:** Why are there times when the baby wakes me up and it's easy for me to get up and there are times that I just can't? Is there an explanation for that?

**A:** The baby wakes up at the end of his or her sleep cycle, but sometimes just as he or she is ending the sleep cycle you are in the deep-sleep stage of your cycle, so you experience difficulty in getting up. This constitutes a severe sleeping disturbance for you.

**Q:** Can we give the baby a meal in his sleep (dream meal) before we go to sleep so that the baby sleeps in late?

**A:** I object to "dream" feeding for three reasons: First, this kind of feeding is dangerous and may lead to a situation called aspiration in which the content of the meal goes into the trachea instead of the esophagus. The baby is unaware of the feeding and that can be dangerous. Second, experience has shown that it does not matter when the baby eats, he or she will usually wake up at the same time and it has to do with the time of sunrise, not the contents of the stomach. And between us, who would want to be fed without feeling it?

**Q:** My friend came to you for sleep coaching and said that you told her that if the baby falls asleep on the breast while breastfeeding it could confuse him or her in learning how to independently fall asleep. Is that true?

**A:** It's certainly true. When the baby nurses and falls asleep on the breast, he or she learns that in order to sleep you don't have to do anything on your own, because the breast will help you. If he or she falls asleep in the stroller, then he or she will want to fall asleep next time while strolling. It's important the baby enters the sleeping process by itself.

**Q:** I am a father to a 5-month-old baby and I feel that I am not doing anything for him when he cries during the learning process for continuous sleep. Can I let him cry for a limited time of one or two minutes?

**A:** When you let your baby cry during the learning process, it does not mean that you are doing nothing. You are certainly doing something. You are allowing him to learn how to fall asleep on his own. It is not advisable to just let the baby cry for no reason, unless it is with a purpose of teaching and acting in accordance with every step of the method.

**Q:** My son is 5 months old and fully breastfeeding. I would very much like to wean him from eating at night and teach him how to sleep but I am concerned that the process will affect the amount of milk that I have. What do I do?

**A:** When you stop breastfeeding at night there is definitely a decrease in production of milk during the baby's sleeping hours. Breastfeeding is a business of supply and demand and if the baby stops breastfeeding at night, milk production will decrease (at night). During the day, while the baby continues to breastfeed at the same frequency and even higher, he will still have as much milk as he needs. There is also the possibility (not as good, in my opinion) of pumping during the night when the baby is sleeping and keeping it to feed him when needed.

# Epilogue and Thanks

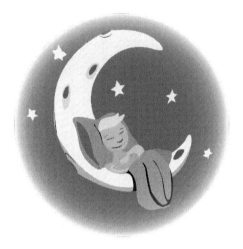

The book that you have just read is a summary of an old love of mine: sleep.

I love to sleep. I need sleep. For me it has never been a waste of time and I am at my best only when I sleep nine hours a night. During the days that I could not sleep those hours, like when I was urgently called to the delivery room, I was less patient with myself and others. My productivity was lower compared to the days I had enough sleep. When people ask me where I get the energy to do so many things, I say, "I sleep nine hours a night."

I am also a mother and putting the children to bed was to part ways after an entire day during which I gave them all of my attention. The moment I had put them in their beds I felt, on the one hand, that this is what they needed, but at the same time, that maybe they needed me to stay with them. When I had attempted to stay with them I found that I was only getting in the way of their falling asleep, but guilt and ambivalence made me act from an emotional rather than a rational place.

I would like to thank from the bottom of my heart the hundreds of couples who chose the "Shhh...at Night We Sleep" method to teach their babies and children to sleep. My heart was especially warmed by those who returned with the second and third and even fourth child, despite the fact that they knew the method. They wanted the supervision and the service that made me feel the method works. I also appreciate all the couples who sent their neighbors and friends with a great desire for more families to get back their sleep.

Thank you to my amazing and professional coaches who are so dedicated. Thank you for helping me spread the method, for teaching more and more babies to sleep a full night. Without you, I would not have found the time to write this book.

I want to send my deepest gratitude to Mrs. Tilly Levine, the woman who urged that this book be translated and published in English. Tilly insisted to do the work fast so that not only her grandchildren will get the opportunity to sleep through the night using the method, but that all children will develop with good health and great happiness. Thank you Tilly, for your love, friendship, wonderful comments and unlimited help.

Thank you to Ms. Cynthia Phillips who believed in me and in my book from our very first meeting. Thank you for your professional and dedicated work. Thank you to Pablo Boyanovsky

Bazan for his wonderful artwork that illustrates the method accurately. Thank you to Mr. Avi Zakori for the helpful and wise comments. Thank you to Mrs. Tali Shilon for the translation from Hebrew to English. Thank you to the wonderful Blair O'Neil for editorial support and book layout.

Thank you to Connie Nelson for joining with enthusiasm towards the end of the project and guiding me. Thank you to the amazing baby Cruz Diaz, who learned to sleep a whole night using my method and is the hero of the cover of the book.

Thank you to Amy and Orlando for the support, encouragement, and help. Thank you to my special children: Shir, Eitay and Rona who help spread the method at every opportunity and connected me with more and more friends who want to sleep.... And a final thank you to Doron my husband, the love of my life. Thank you for the support, help and partnership in our personal and professional life. Thank you for not snoring and letting me sleep.

And thank you, dear parents, for purchasing this book. I don't just believe that you will succeed in teaching your babies and children to sleep with it, I KNOW that you will succeed! Yes, you can!

It is wonderful that I may be able to make up for my personal experience with my children through you, dear parents, who will teach your children to sleep. Just sleep.

In friendship and love,
Dorit Kreiser

# Appendixes and Addendums

**Appendix A:**
**Sleep Hours by Age**

| Age | # of Hours/24 | # of hours during daytime |
|---|---|---|
| Birth-3 months | 16-18 | All throughout the day |
| 3-6 months | 15-18 | 3 sleep periods during the day |
| 6-9 months | 15 | 3 sleep periods during the day |
| 9-12 months | 15 | 2 sleep periods during the day |
| 12-18 months | 13 | Once a day (an hour-and-a-half) |
| 18-24 months | 13 | Once a day (an hour-and-a-half) |
| 2-3.5 years | 12 | Once a day (an hour-and-a-half) |
| 3.5 – 5 years | 12 | Most kids don't need to sleep during The day, but it is recommended to have an hour a day with little to no stimulation |

## Appendix B:
## Scientific Research in the Field of Sleep and Related Issues

Claude Lenfant. The interdependence of sleep and health – A commentary. Metabolism – Clinical and Experimental, 2006, 55: S50-s53.[LE27]

Cochrane Database System Rev. (April, 2017) Infant pacifiers for reduction in risk of sudden infant death syndrome

Dahl, R. E., & Harvey, A. G. (2007). Sleep in children and adolescents with behavioral and emotional disorders. Sleep Medicine Clinics, 2, 503 Ferber, R. (2006). Solve your child's sleep problems (Rev ed.). London, England: Dorling Kindersley

Huber, R. & Born, J. (2014). Sleep, Synaptic Connectivity, and Hippocampal memory during early development. March 2014 vol. 18, no. 3

Jan, J. E., Reiter, R. J., Bax, M. C. O., Ribary, U., Freeman, R. D., & Wasdell, M. B. (2010). Long-termsleep disturbances in children: A cause of neuronal loss. European Journal of Pediatric Neurology, 14, 380–388

Janet M., Mullington, Monika, H., Toth, M., Jorge, M. S. & Hans K. (2009). Meier-Ewers Cardiovascular, Inflammatory, and Metabolic Consequences of Sleep Deprivation. Progress in cardiovascular diseases, Vol. 51 ,no. 4 (January & February). pp. 294-302 Lee, E. K., & Douglass, A. B. (2010). Sleep in psychiatric disorders: Where are we now? The Canadian Journal of Psychiatry, 55, 408–412

Malhotra, A. & Loscalzo, J. (2009) Sleep and cardiovascular disease: An overview. Progress in Cardiovascular Diseases. 51 (4), 279-284

Maslow, A. H. (1943). A theory of human motivation. Psychological Review. Originally published in Psychological Review, 50, 370-396

Mathias Basner,Kenneth M. Fomberstein; Farid M.Razavil et al. American Time Use Survey: Sleep

Time and its Relationship to Waking Activities. Sleep, 2007, 30: 1085-1090.

Meijer, A. M., & van den Wittenboer, G. L. H. (2007). Contribution of infants' sleep and crying to marital relationship of first-time parent couples in the 1st year after childbirth. Journal of Family Psychology, 21, 49–53

Michael A. Grandner, Nirav P. Patel, Philip R. Gehrman, et al. Problems associated with short sleep: Bridging the gap between laboratory and epidemiological studies. Sleep Medicine Reviews, 2010, 14: 240-247

Mindell, J. A., Kuhn, B. R., Lewin, D. S., Meltzer, L. J., & Sadeh, A. (2006). Behavioral treatment of bedtime problems and night walkings in infants and young children. Sleep, 29, 1263–1270. Retrieved from http://www.journalsleep.org

Nunes, M. L., & Bruni, O. (2015). Insomnia in childhood and adolescence: Clinical aspects, diagnosis, and therapeutic approach. Journal de Pediatria, (305), 1-10 Peter Meerlo,Andrea Sgoifo,Deborah Suchecki. Restricted and disrupted sleep:Effects on autonomic function, neuroendocrine stress systems and stress responsivity. Sleep Medicine Reviews, 2008, 12: 197-210.

Stickgold, R., Hobson, J. A., Fosse, R. & Fosse, M. (2001). Sleep, learning, and dreams: Off-line memory reprocessing. Science 294 (5544):1052–57 Tomas, J. H., Moor, M. & Mindell, J.A. (2014). Controversies in behavioral treatment of sleep problems in young children Sleep. Medicine clinic. 9, 251-259

Psaila K et al, Infant pacifiers for Reduction in Risk of Sudden Infant Death Syndrome. Cochrane Database Syst Rev. (April, 2017)

Made in the USA
Middletown, DE
01 August 2021

45160630R00137